Finally, a holistic approach to healing from a qualified physician who has both the personal and professional experience to document it. In this book Dr. Rita Hancock integrates the study of the body, the soul, and the spirit, respecting the disciplines of each profession, yet finding the connection within each that offers healing.

—KERRY SHOOK
COAUTHOR OF *ONE MONTH TO LIVE: THIRTY DAYS TO
A NO-REGRETS LIFE* AND *LOVE AT LAST SIGHT: THIRTY
DAYS TO DEEPEN YOUR CLOSEST RELATIONSHIPS*

As a professor and licensed mental health counselor I have seen students and clients struggle with emotional and spiritual issues. These issues can have severe physical consequences that can greatly accentuate the emotional and spiritual underpinnings. Dr. Rita Hancock's book offers the client a positive and long-lasting way out with the process of inner healing and solid Christian-based counseling. Having incorporated inner healing into my own work with traumatized clients, I see Dr. Hancock's book as a refreshing and positive reminder that with the power of God we can be fully healed.

—BENJAMIN B. KEYES, PHD, EDD
PROFESSOR/PROGRAM DIRECTOR, MASTERS IN COUNSELING
REGENT UNIVERSITY

I am excited to see how Dr. Hancock is incorporating forgiveness and inner healing into her pain practice, exposing her clients to a complete body, soul, and spirit healing. I am thankful for her forerunning in joining these practices to give her patients the best help possible. I expect to hear of many more pain-free clients coming from this practice!

—DAWNA DESILVA
FOUNDER AND COLEADER OF SOZO MINISTRY
BETHEL CHURCH
REDDING, CA

D1407979

RADICAL
WELL-BEING

RADICAL
WELL-BEING

RITA HANCOCK, MD

SILOAM

RADICAL WELL-BEING by Rita Hancock, MD
Published by Siloam
Charisma Media/Charisma House Book Group
600 Rinehart Road
Lake Mary, Florida 32746
www.charismahouse.com

Unless otherwise noted, all Scripture quotations are from the Holy Bible, New International Version. Copyright © 1973, 1978, 1984, International Bible Society. Used by permission.

Scripture quotations marked AMP are from the Amplified Bible. Old Testament copyright © 1965, 1987 by the Zondervan Corporation. The Amplified New Testament copyright © 1954, 1958, 1987 by the Lockman Foundation. Used by permission.

Scripture quotations marked ESV are from the Holy Bible, English Standard Version. Copyright © 2001 by Crossway Bibles, a division of Good News Publishers. Used by permission.

Scripture quotations marked KJV are from the King James Version of the Bible.

Scripture quotations marked NKJV are from the New King James Version of the Bible. Copyright © 1979, 1980, 1982 by Thomas Nelson, Inc., publishers. Used by permission.

Scripture quotations marked NLT are from the Holy Bible, New Living Translation, copyright © 1996, 2004, 2007. Used by permission of Tyndale House Publishers, Inc., Wheaton, IL 60189. All rights reserved.

Published in association with the literary agency of WordServe Literary Group, Ltd., 10152 S. Knoll Circle, Highlands Ranch, CO 80130.

Cover design by Justin Evans
Design Director: Bill Johnson

Visit the author's website at www.RadicalWell-Being.com.

Library of Congress Cataloging-in-Publication Data:
An application to register this book for cataloging has been submitted to
the Library of Congress.
International Standard Book Number: 978-1-61638-973-4
E-book ISBN: 978-1-62136-000-1

First edition

13 14 15 16 17 — 987654321
Printed in the United States of America

CONTENTS

Acknowledgments xi
Introduction xiii

PART ONE
"YOU'RE NO GOOD"
Bad Old Lies and What They Do to You

Chapter 1: Don't Believe Everything You Think. 1
Chapter 2: Trace Your Triggers 11
Chapter 3: Stress Less, Betty. 20

PART TWO
THE WHOLE YOU
Connecting Mind, Body, and Spirit

Chapter 4: A Whole in Three. 31
Chapter 5: New Hope for Pain Sufferers 43
Chapter 6: Sometimes Your Senses Lie. 61

PART THREE
THE SPIRITUAL YOU
Seeing Through God's Eyes

Chapter 7: The Accuser 73
Chapter 8: You Are Delightful 83
Chapter 9: No More Judgment. 93

PART FOUR
TAKE CAPTIVE EVERY THOUGHT
How Right Thinking Leads to Right Actions

Chapter 10: Taking Control 105
Chapter 11: No Comparisons 118
Chapter 12: Have No Fear! 123

Chapter 13: Power Plays 132
Chapter 14: Reject Perfectionism. 140
Chapter 15: Managing Family Strife. 149
Chapter 16: Filtering Out Lies in Advertising. 158
Chapter 17: Confession and Repentance Set You Free. 168
Chapter 18: Forgiveness Sets *You* Free 178

PART FIVE

HOPE IN YOUR FUTURE

Biblical Steps to Healing and Health

Chapter 19: Introduction to Inner Healing 191
Chapter 20: Inner Healing in My Unique Medical Practice. 204
Chapter 21: Let God Speak Into Your Imagination 215
Chapter 22: Choose Truth Over Lies 223
Chapter 23: Your True Identity 232

Conclusion 242
Appendix A: Praying for Emotional Healing. 244
Appendix B: Scripture for Self-Talk and Meditation 248
Notes 255
About the Author. 259
Index 260

Acknowledgments

If it weren't for God, who created me and all the people whose stories I melded into this book, I would have no life, no love, and, most certainly, no book. So first and foremost, thank You, God.

Second, thank you to my husband, Ed, the man who led me to Christ. When we were first married, Ed didn't push me toward God. He just remained cool and peaceful and made me want what he had.

Thank you to our children, Lindsey and Cory, who inspire me and whose existence showed me the nature of love. I delight in them, just as God delights in us.

Thank you to my physician-mentors for equipping me with the nuts and bolts of medicine.

Thank you to my patients, who showed me how to artfully put the nuts and bolts together.

Thank you to my manual medicine family: Dr. Ed Stiles, Micha, Holly, Steve, Kay, Margo, Dr. Ross Pope, and many, many others. Without you I wouldn't feel as good as I do personally or have the magnified skills to heal others through the mind, body, and spirit.

Thank you to my pastor, Craig Groeschel, and other pastors of LifeChurch.tv, who encourage people to find and develop their unique spiritual gifts and start new ministries.

Last, and certainly not least, thank you to my agent, Greg Johnson, and the editors and staff at Charisma House, including Debbie Marrie, Woodley Auguste, Althea Thompson, Atalie Anderson, Justin Evans, Adrienne Gaines, Leigh DeVore, and everyone else who helped make this book a reality. As the saying goes, "It takes a village to raise a child." From what I've seen, it also takes a village to write a book.

*"Behold, You desire truth in the inner being;
make me therefore to know wisdom in my inmost heart."*
—PSALM 51:6, AMP

INTRODUCTION

SOME PEOPLE THINK doctors can't relate to the problems of the average Jane or Joe. If that's the case, I don't fit into the usual doctor mold. When I was a little girl, I was morbidly obese. I don't have to tell you how that can affect a child's self-esteem and emotions. Probably you already know.

Through most of elementary school I weighed double what the "normal" kids weighed, mostly because I ate huge portions of food and ate too often, without regard to actual physical hunger. I also consumed large volumes of sugary, high-calorie soda pop and watched too much television. Instead of sitting on my bottom and eating, I should have been outside, running around and playing.

Anytime I felt bored, anxious, angry, frustrated, or sad, I ate. One of my favorite emotional pick-me-ups was to put a dozen Chips Ahoy cookies in a large bowl, pour milk over the cookies, and eat the soggy concoction like it was a bowl of cereal.

Not surprisingly, for my first-ever job I worked as a "doughnut finisher" at Dunkin' Donuts. That means I filled and frosted the doughnuts the bakers made. Within six months of starting that job, I "finished" enough doughnuts to gain another twenty pounds. I topped off at over 207 pounds, and I was only seventeen years old and only five feet tall.

As you can imagine, I hated the way I felt because of my obesity. Throughout school I was always the last kid picked for sports teams, and I was frequently teased and bullied because of my weight.

Thankfully, the sad story of my childhood obesity has a happy ending. In my young adult life I discovered the secret to taking off the excess weight and keeping it off, and it had nothing to do with dieting or willpower. It had to do with correcting the underlying thoughts and beliefs that led to my weight gain to begin with.

Before I go on, let me clarify what this book is about. Even though my personal battle was with obesity, this isn't just a weight-loss book. This is a total health book. I tell you not only how to triumph over obesity but also how to triumph over chronic pain, stress-induced illness, depression, anxiety, anger, drug and alcohol abuse, and other types of physical, spiritual, and emotional bondage.

Even if your outlet is different from mine (i.e., if you take drugs, drink alcohol, or compulsively shop or gamble instead of overeat), you and I probably have a few things in common. We fall into addictive behaviors in our attempts to escape the emotions that secretly bug us deep down.

Hear me, now, because I am trying to help you. Your real enemy is not the bad habit or illness you're focused on getting rid of, whether it's overeating, alcoholism, chronic pain, or some other vice. Your real enemy lies deeper than your surface behavior, in the invisible, spiritual realm as well as in your subconscious mind.

Because of whatever went on in your life when you were a child, you might have internalized false beliefs into your subconscious mind, such as "I'm worthless," "I'm bad," "It's my fault," "I'm stupid," "I'm weak," "I'm just like my bad (mother or father), "(He, she, or it) is my responsibility," "I'm dirty," "I'm shameful," "I'm ugly," and so on. You probably even carried those lies with you into your adult life.

Fast-forward to today, and new circumstances in your life stir up those old, internalized lies and resultant unpleasant emotions from childhood. Reliving those old, unpleasant emotions seems unbearable, so you reflexively seek solace in drugs, alcohol, food, sex, or the pursuit of money to get your mind off of how you feel. Or you literally transform your unwanted emotions into pain and/or stress-induced illness so you don't have to be aware of them consciously.

If I just described you, don't worry. I have good news that will bring you relief. It's actually *the* good news. God's truth sets you free from all of it: the lies, the unwanted emotions, the unwanted behaviors, and the stress-induced illnesses that result from those emotions.

Get it? Through this book I help you get to the root of your problem and correct it at its source rather than rely on willpower alone to control your outward behavior. It takes less energy to do it that way (because it's God's energy and not yours), and it gives you longer-lasting relief too.

Becoming an Expert

It had to be the grace of God that allowed me to lose seventy-five pounds by the end of high school, right before leaving for college at Cornell University. I say that because I didn't actually know a thing about nutrition or health at the time I actually lost the weight. All I did was eat less, give up sugary soda pop, give up TV, and exercise more. It just seemed logical, and it worked.

When I got to Cornell, I minored in nutrition and grew more and more determined to do everything I could to keep the weight off. I figured more knowledge was better, and Ivy League nutrition knowledge was therefore best.

Unfortunately I was wrong. Memorizing nutritional biochemistry pathways and minutia such as how much beta-carotene is in a sweet potato didn't help me control my weight at all. If anything, I think it made matters worse. The more I knew about what was in the food, the more obsessed I became about what I ate. I even developed a compulsive eating disorder by my sophomore year, because studying nutrition minutia just fed my obsession in the wrong way.

Thanks to God (even though I didn't actually know Him yet), I began to find relief from my eating disorder fairly quickly. By my junior year God led me to a faculty advisor in the area of obesity psychology. Between his wisdom and what I learned from secular, self-help, anti-dieting books, I realized that I had been using food as an emotional crutch.

After graduation from Cornell, I went to medical school at the State University of New York at Buffalo, during which time I was awarded research fellowships in nutrition and digestive diseases, including a prestigious fellowship funded by the National Institutes of Health for selected medical students. Eventually I became a board-certified physical medicine and rehabilitation specialist and a board-certified subspecialist in pain management.

Though I've been in practice for nearly sixteen years, the last eight or nine years have been the best by far. That's because during that time I stopped treating patients with addictive narcotic painkillers and started using osteopathic manual medicine (OMM) to alleviate pain in a more natural way.

OMM is a hands-on manipulation technique that can involve gently helping the patient to bend, twist, and turn in order to unwind tension from the person's tissues and restore normal flexibility. It can also involve high-velocity popping techniques, but I like the gentle, indirect techniques better.

For the most part I learned OMM from Ed Stiles, DO, and his primary Oklahoma protégé, Micha Sale, PT, as well as my own OMM physician, Ross Pope, DO, and a number of other PT experts in Micha's entourage too numerous to mention.

So you can understand the level of OMM teaching I've been blessed to receive, let me say that in 2009 Dr. Stiles won the A. T. Still Award, which is the highest honor in the *world* in the area of osteopathic manual medicine! Do you know how Hollywood has the Oscars, but each year one actor or actress receives the Lifetime Achievement Award? That's how big the A. T. Still Award is in the area of osteopathic manual medicine. It's like a lifetime achievement award. That's why I see myself as being exceptionally blessed by God. I have had the mind-boggling luxury of having nearly two hundred fifty hours of instruction with the famous Dr. Ed Stiles, not to mention another five hundred hours at least with Micha, who can out-OMM most DOs out there from what I've seen.

The best part of learning Dr. Stiles's methods is the side-effect of emotional healing that I can now offer my patients. Thanks to the special dialoguing language that he taught me, I am much better able to relate to my patients on a deep, emotional level that fosters quick and permanent healing. In turn I am more able to help my patients overcome not only pain but also stress-induced illnesses and addictions.

But, again, let me give credit where credit is due. It wasn't my studying, research, and hands-on training with doctors and physical therapists that changed my life. It was the grace of God Himself, who orchestrated the events of my life to come together in this exact way. Without Him I wouldn't have found my own personal healing, and I wouldn't be offering the same to you.

The Next Chapter in My Life

During my years of having babies and trying to balance motherhood with my busy doctor schedule, I encountered new difficulties maintaining my weight. Again, thankfully, I was able to drop the pregnancy weight and get back to my current, comfortable weight of about 132 pounds.

Why was I able to keep the weight off when so many others fail at weight control? I believe it's because God helped me to identify the real reasons I gained the weight as a child.

When I gave my life to God about ten years ago, He markedly accelerated my emotional healing—well beyond the relief I gained from intellectual knowledge alone back in college. He magnified my understanding so I could experience the fruit of the Spirit in a more general sense. He revealed the truth about why I reached for false comforters instead of Him, including the lies I believed about myself and my sin. That knowledge set me free, just as Scripture talks about in John 8:31-32 (NKJV).

> Then Jesus said to those Jews who believed Him, "If you abide in My word, you are My disciples indeed. And you shall know the truth, and the truth shall make you free."

I pray that as you read through this book you experience the same sort of acceleration in emotional healing that I've been able to experience by His grace. That way you can shed your need for your false comforters, just as I have.

Hope for Healing

I am a pain-management doctor. Many of the patients I see have pain due to muscle, nerve, spine, and joint problems. Being that I live in Oklahoma (the sixth most obese state in the nation), most of my patients are also overweight. And because my patients are human, most have some degree of emotional baggage that makes their pain seem even worse.

To help my patients I offer spinal and soft tissue injections, electrical nerve tests, OMM, and non-narcotic pain medicines. However, I also address my patients' deep-down emotional stressors that magnify their pain and increase their suffering. I believe in the mind-body-spirit connection, and you can't treat the whole person by focusing only on the physical being.

Perhaps you are like my patients and have spine or joint pain or some other stress-induced physical illness such as fibromyalgia, irritable bowel syndrome, migraines, ulcers, or high blood pressure. Relieving your emotional stress can, at the minimum, lessen the intensity of your symptoms. In some cases it can eliminate your discomfort entirely.

Perhaps you also seek to lessen or eliminate stress-induced and addictive behaviors such as overeating, smoking, alcoholism, shopping, porn, or gambling. I like to call these things "false comforters" because they help you only in the short-term. In the long-term they consume you and destroy your finances, your physical health, and your relationships.

No matter why you were led to this book, your real key to freedom involves going deeper than you realize. Dig under your surface symptom (the drugs, alcohol, shopping, food, etc.) and find the deep-down lies that triggered you to reach for the false comfort in the first place. Once you eliminate the emotional stress at its source, the physical problems and bad behaviors lessen on their own.

How This Book Is Laid Out

I have divided this book into five parts. The first, "You're No Good," shows how lies we learned about ourselves as children can affect us as adults. We may attach judgment, self-condemnation, and shame to our false beliefs. Through emotional triggers present-day events cause us to tap into those old lies we have believed and lead us to damaging behaviors as we search for emotional consolation.

In The Whole You I introduce you to a new perspective on physical health. Controlling your unwanted behavior is important, but it's *not* the whole answer. Good health requires paying attention to the inter-relationship between mind, body, and spirit.

Your answers start with your submitting your mind to God. The Spiritual You shows that rather than listen to the lies of the accuser, you must allow the Lord to reframe how you think. Your Creator loves you so much that He died for you.

In Taking Every Thought Captive I talk about how managing your thought life is a critical part of your long-term health. Then in Hope in Your Future I detail practical, biblical steps you can take—such as repentance, forgiveness, Christian counseling, prayer, and relying on God's Word—to promote healing and better health not just for today but also for the rest of your life.

Finally in the appendixes I provide you with resources to augment your healing through Scripture-based mind renewal.

Are You Eager to Get Started?

Are you at the point where you're sick and tired of wasting time, money, and mental energy on your problems? Are you finally willing to dig deeper into the emotions and subconscious lies that trigger your unhealthy behavior rather than simply cover up your problem with temporary false comfort? Are you willing to get real with yourself?

By the time patients get to me for their pain and weight problems, they are generally exhausted and ready for deep-down help. I imagine you are too, or you wouldn't have picked up this book.

My friend, I praise God for your faith and courage! And I pray that your continued reading is blessed with supernatural clarity and recep-tiveness so that you can feel the same emotional freedom I have expe-rienced, as well as find relief from your unwanted addictive behaviors, physical pain, and stress-induced illness.

PART ONE

"YOU'RE NO GOOD"

BAD OLD LIES AND WHAT THEY DO TO YOU

Chapter 1

DON'T BELIEVE
EVERYTHING YOU THINK

I F I ASKED you to look at a group of women and pick out the person with the eating disorder, you wouldn't choose Helen. She doesn't fit the stereotype. She's a slightly overweight, sixty-year-old grandmother. Surprise! Not all people with eating disorders are skinny, teenage girls.

As I interviewed Helen about her knee pain on that first medical visit, she repeatedly pointed out that she was desperate to lose weight so her knees would hurt less. On the surface that made sense. However, something wasn't right about this particular situation. She seemed more fixated on the prospect of weight loss than on relieving the knee pain.

That's when she starting asking me about my previous book, *The Eden Diet*. Apparently her daughter had lost a fair amount of weight on the diet, and Helen now wanted to try it.

I have to admit that I was a little confused by this point in the visit. She was on the schedule as wanting to be seen for her knees. So I just came out and asked, "Shouldn't we be talking about your knees?"

Helen looked down at the ground and then back up at me. "Well, I heard you don't see just anybody for weight loss. I heard you mostly treat pain-management patients and just counsel them for weight loss on the side. I guess I figured that you could help me kill two birds with one stone."

You have to commend her persistence. That's faith and desperation rolled into one! I figured I'd better help her or she'd get some people to take the shingles off the roof of my office and lower her into the exam room through the ceiling on a stretcher while thinking, "If only I touch the hem of her lab coat, I'll lose weight."

As Helen and I dialogued in subsequent visits, I gleaned some insight into her underlying problem. As a child she internalized lies that led her into an eating disorder in her teenage years. She believed her mother would love her only if she was skinny. Her mother had been a dancer in her youth and pressured Helen and her sisters to not eat too much or they wouldn't be wanted (by men). But Helen understood that nobody, not even her own mother, would want her if she were overweight.

Hence the eating disorder. She was trying to "works" her way into being good enough by manipulating (or trying to manipulate) her weight. Hidden lies and feelings of inadequacy, such as those Helen entertained, lead to emotional stress and strife. In turn those lies lead to overeating and other physical manifestations, such as pain and illness. It's a common tale, one that another of my patients knows well.

A Little Girl Named Nancy

Nancy's parents rarely had time for her. Her father was an attorney in a big Chicago law firm, and if he didn't work long hours, he wouldn't stand a chance of becoming partner. Based on his own standards for success, that would have meant he was a total failure in life. He learned that way of thinking from his dad, who was also a highly successful, perfectionist, workaholic lawyer with low self-esteem deep down.

Nancy's mother was a legal secretary in the same firm. She didn't have to work overtime with her husband all those evenings, but she did so anyway, saying it was to help her husband get home earlier. Truthfully she just wanted to keep tabs on her good-looking, wealthy husband. She didn't trust him around the perky little legal interns.

The one source of constancy in Nancy's early life was her paternal grandfather. He babysat her most evenings after day care or school when her parents worked overtime, and he watched her most Saturdays too. The babysitting job kept him from getting lonely and depressed since his wife had passed away a few years before. Without the pairing, both he and Nancy would have been alone.

Despite Nancy's company, Grandpa was still lonely in a different kind of way. To fill that need, he fell into reading inappropriate magazines. He made a halfhearted attempt to hide the magazines from little Nancy but failed. She found them by accident one day shortly after her seventh birthday while looking for magazine pictures she could use for a school art project.

A flurry of questions ran through her little mind when she found those pictures. "Why would Grandpa look at those magazines? Is this how men are supposed to look at women? Is this how women are supposed to be looked at?"

Though Nancy was young, she knew instinctively that her grandpa's magazines were naughty, and she felt bad about herself for having seen them. In fact, she experienced not just a single crush but a double crush to her self-esteem over this.

On one hand she couldn't help but identify with the women in the pictures. If they were just lowly objects, then maybe that's all she was too. After all, she was female, just like them. On the other hand, Nancy identified with her grandfather and felt deep shame. "Grandpa is bad for looking at these," she thought, "so I must be bad too, because we're related and that means I'm like him."

The blow to her self-esteem stayed with her for a long time, compromising her romantic relationships with men later in life. She couldn't trust them. Were they looking at her as a piece of meat or as a person? Would they betray her as her daddy betrayed her mommy? Or would they abandon her as her parents abandoned her to focus on their work? She was never sure.

This incident also marked the beginning of her overeating. On a subconscious level, seeing those pictures at that impressionable age caused Nancy to feel vulnerable and out of control in addition to bad and dirty. Nancy decided she didn't want anyone to look at her the way her grandfather looked at those women. So she ate to put a layer of insulation around her body. It backfired, though, because people looked anyway since she was so large.

This issue with her grandfather wasn't the only reason Nancy gained weight as a child. On some level, even though her daddy ultimately made partner in the firm and was able to spend more time at home, Nancy always felt a sense of abandonment due to his earlier absence. She figured that she was unworthy of Daddy's attention. If she were a good enough daughter, maybe he would have stayed home.

These feelings of low self-esteem and abandonment gave her another reason to eat to keep people away as an adult. If nobody became interested in her romantically because she was overweight, then nobody would abandon or betray her later on.

Of course, during her childhood Nancy was totally unaware of these buried feelings. It wasn't until she underwent counseling to save her third failing marriage that she began to understand the psychology that motivated her to eat as a child.

Through counseling, Nancy learned that she felt shameful, vulnerable, and out of control as a child, especially sexually but also emotionally. Eating was her unconscious attempt to feel safe and in control. She ate to medicate her low self-esteem and anxiety, and she ate to keep away unwanted attention.

Composite Patients

Can you relate to any part of Helen's or Nancy's story? They actually represent composites of a multitude of women whom I've counseled for weight loss, pain, and other stress-related health problems over the years. In fact, all the patient examples that I present in this book are composites—yet every situation I describe is real.

As you can see by Helen's and Nancy's examples, fear, sexuality, and feeling inadequate or out of control are common themes that contribute to aberrant eating behavior in women. Other common issues include guilt, low self-esteem, abandonment or loss (such as parental divorce), parental alcoholism, and physical illness during childhood. Because I hear these themes frequently in my medical practice, you'll see them often in the patient composites I include in this book.

My intent in presenting these composites is to help you understand

and manage your emotional triggers and, consequently, have an easier time letting go of your addictions, unwanted behaviors, and physical pain. Even better than the physical benefits, though, is the peace, love, and joy you feel when you break free from false beliefs and feel more of the fruit of the Spirit in your life. I assure you that the freedom from emotional bondage feels even better than the physical health benefits.

The Lies That Bind

In the following pages I list fundamental beliefs that have triggered feelings of stress, depression, and anxiety in some of my patients. In many cases the emotions caused by these beliefs led my patients to reach for false comforters (food, alcohol, gambling, spending, over-working, etc.) to try to feel better.

Before you read the list, please pray. (See Appendix A for more help with prayer.) Ask God to reveal only the information that you can handle, and ask Him to reveal if you should dig through these subconscious beliefs with the help of a Christian counselor. Not everyone is meant to "go there" without the help of another human. God gave us Christian counselors and psychologists for a reason.

Now if the time is right (and only you and God can be the judge of that, so proceed at your own risk and do so prayerfully), read the list and see if any of the lies strike a nerve. Make a checkmark by each one that does.

Keep in mind that *everything* on the bulleted list is a lie. Even though you see the accusations against you in print, don't be fooled into believing them.

- You're fat.
- You're ugly.
- You're stupid.
- You're unlovable.
- God doesn't love you.
- You're bad (or not good enough).

- You're worthless.

- You'll never amount to anything.

- You shouldn't have been born.

- They're going to leave you.

- You don't deserve to be loved.

- It's all your fault.

- You're dirty.

- You're shameful.

- It's your fault your parents divorced.

- You're unforgivable because of the abortion.

- You're a bad mother for giving up your baby when you were a teenager.

- If you were worth anything, she wouldn't have given you up for adoption.

- Your parents adopted you to fix their marriage; now their happiness is up to you.

- If you were good, your dad (or mom) would have stuck around.

- It's your fault your mom or dad drank.

- It's your fault your dad abused your mom (or vice versa).

- It's your fault he sexually abused you.

- You deserve to be treated badly.

- She'll never let your daddy hear the last of it if you tell on him.

- Your mother won't believe you if you tell her about the abuse.

- It's your fault he (or she) left.

- It's your fault he (or she) died.

- You're just like your bad mother.

- You're just like your bad father.

- You're not as good as your brother or sister.

- You're an accident.

- You weren't wanted.

- You can't be forgiven for what you did.

- They're going to leave you if they find out you're bad.

- You have to try to be perfect to make up for being bad.

- You don't deserve anybody's time.

- God's promises aren't meant for you.

Remember, these are lies that have nothing to do with who you are today. It's important to identify the beliefs that you learned in the past, as we will see. Realize that the time has come to let go of the lies, and I help you do that in this book. Now let's talk about other sources of false childhood beliefs.

Lies That Make You *Think* You're Fat

Because my daughter is a teenager, I spend a fair amount of time watching the effects of peer pressure on the kids in her age group. Even the more wholesome TV programs that are geared to her age group show perfectly manicured, extremely cute girls with perfect clothing and most excellent hair. Naturally, real-life girls of that age group are bound to feel inadequate.

I know about peer pressure for another reason. I temporarily volunteered my services to online "ask the expert" websites. I quit after having to answer the same anonymous question a thousand times from teenage girls: "Dr. Rita, please tell me how to lose thirty pounds in the next three weeks. I'm going to be in my sister's wedding, and I'm a total blimp. I'm over one hundred thirty pounds, and I'm only five foot seven inches. I want to get down to the same weight as the other bridesmaids."

How did I respond? "Honey, your real problem isn't your weight. You may have an eating disorder. You should talk with your parents and get some counseling."

I wish I could have spoken freely about my faith to those girls on that secular site. If I had been able to, I would have said, "No matter how hard you try, you will never be somebody else, and you will never feel that you're good enough after you lose weight if you feel inadequate before. Your greatest journey is to get in line with God's will for your life, not to get in line with God's will for somebody else's life."

Thinking you're fat eventually makes you become fat. Your actions affect your attitudes, and your attitudes affect your actions. Watch what you think because it will affect what you do.

You Have to Ask the Questions

If you aren't sure about what triggers you to reach for false comforters, start asking questions: "Immediately before I feel tempted to [eat, drink, gamble, shop, overwork, etc.], do I feel fear, anger, or low self-esteem? Do I feel stupid, worthless, or out of control? Or do I feel unnurtured? Or is it something else?

"And how do I feel *after* I utilize my false comforter? Do those emotions go away? If so, for how long do they go away?" As I said, the false comforter is *not* the underlying problem. It's only the attempted solution to get away from the unwanted emotion.

Many people feel out of control and hence, fearful or anxious. They use their false comforters to try to regain a sense of control. "Nobody can tell me what to [eat, buy, smoke, drink, feel, etc.]." Or they use the false comforters as short-term distractions to escape their emotions. They cover their anger, fear, or low self-esteem with alcohol, drugs, food, shopping, cutting, or some other unhealthy behavior.

The Right Questions Break Down Barriers

Surveying and assessing your emotions can definitely help you identify your triggers. However, it's even better to petition the all-knowing Creator of the universe for answers. He knows the nature of your deep-down issues better than you do!

You may be thinking, "But I've asked Him for answers a million times, and He doesn't answer!" If you feel as if God isn't answering you, or if you feel "lost" in your journey for answers, realize the problem isn't likely to be on God's end. You may have barriers that prevent you from hearing from God.

Many factors can serve as barriers that block your reception of God's healing. For example, maybe you believe lies about yourself as a result of childhood events or abuse. Or maybe you need to repent of past sins. Maybe you need to extend forgiveness to those who hurt you. Maybe you are mad at God because you couldn't find Him during your times of trouble. Maybe you feel ashamed and are hiding from God. Or maybe it's something entirely different. Maybe you have emotional or physical barriers.

No matter what caused your barriers to go up, asking God the *right* questions about the nature of those barriers can help to tear them down.

To help you overcome your barriers, at the ends of the chapters in Parts 1–4 I offer sample questions that you can ask God during prayer. To formulate these questions, I borrowed from a number of healing disciplines, including Christian inner-healing ministry, psychology, physical therapy, and manual medicine, all of which talk about overcoming barriers of one form or another. That way, once your barriers come down, you can better receive healing truth from God and, in turn, experience freedom from your emotional triggers and bondage to false comforters.

ACTION POINT
Ask God in Prayer

⚬ Express your thankfulness and confidence: "Dear Lord, thank You for the healing truth that I am about to receive."

⚬ Ask for a new start: "As I recall my past sins, please forgive me, wash me clean, and make me brand-new."

⚬ Ask God to help you drop your defenses: "Lord, please amplify my ability to hear and/or understand deep healing truth as I read."

⚬ Ask for compassion: "Lord, please help me to have compassion toward myself and others. Help me forgive those who hurt me."

Chapter 2

TRACE YOUR TRIGGERS

I N THE FIRST few years after I started treating Rebeca, she was in the office nearly every few weeks with a new pain complaint. Yet when I reviewed her physical exam, imaging studies, and blood work, I found no actual cause for her pain. She didn't even have muscles spasms, alignment problems, or fibromyalgia. That's why I probed into the possibility that her pain might be stress-induced.

I had good reason to suspect that emotions were the problem. Rebeca was an only child, and at the age of fifteen (about forty years ago) she lost her mother to cancer. Actually she lost both parents when her mother died, because her father became permanently emotionally shell-shocked by the loss. Basically she was orphaned, even though one parent was still living.

Because of my hunch, the next time Rebeca had a pain attack, I took a different approach than I had in the past. I asked Rebeca to put a name on the emotion she felt at that moment in time. It turned out the word was *afraid*. I then asked her to think back to the very earliest time she felt the same level of fear. I figured there might have been an emotionally charged event in her past that was fueling her present anxiety.

Rebeca looked up at the ceiling for a few seconds, lost in thought. But then her face changed abruptly. On one hand she looked as if she had seen a ghost, but on the other hand she looked excited and happy. She was nearly breathless too. Obviously she remembered something significant related to her present fear. I just couldn't tell if it was good or bad.

It doesn't usually happen this way, but the first word out of Rebeca's mouth was her diagnosis. She said, "Abandonment!" She went on to say, "My husband left for a business trip the day before this new pain attack started!" She connected the dots without my help. She felt just as abandoned as when her mother died.

What's doubly interesting is that within about thirty seconds of her epiphany, her leg pain decreased by almost half. It still hurt, but it was much more tolerable. Notice that I helped her pain without touching her.

Can you relate to Rebeca's story? Have you ever overreacted to a situation and then in hindsight said, "Why on earth did such a small thing affect me so intensely?" Perhaps a present-day trigger—a smell, a sight, a sound, a thought—tapped into a past experience that was infused with negative emotion such as fear.

You perceive your present circumstances through the lenses of your past experiences. As the saying goes, "We don't see things as they are. We see things as *we* are." In this chapter I show you how events of your past shape your interpretation of present-day events and hence your current emotions. I also demonstrate how children typically misjudge or misinterpret past events to some degree, if for no other reason than because of their inexperience and lack of objectivity relative to adults. Understanding these dynamics in your memories can help you learn how to dialogue with your inner child and proceed toward emotional healing.

Childhood Misperceptions Drive You to False Comforters

Kids see the world through immature minds. Consequently their conclusions and interpretations about traumatic events can be downright warped, if for no other reason than their immaturity and inexperience.

If you're seven years old and daddy sexually abuses you, you might conclude (using your seven-year-old reasoning skills) that there's something wrong with *you* because of it. Obviously that's wrong. But kids see the world and draw conclusions based on what they think they know. Then their wrong conclusions become their reality.

It's too bad we can't psychically know what our kids are thinking in response to childhood shock and trauma so we could correct their thinking earlier rather than later.

In a way, adults aren't much better off than children. No matter how old and experienced we are, we still "see through a glass, darkly," as it says in 1 Corinthians 13:12 (KJV). We can't completely understand things from God's full, objective perspective.

Remember Nancy? During conflicts in her adult life she practiced avoidance due to the fear of abandonment that she developed in childhood. Back then she internalized certain beliefs, not knowing they were false. As a child Nancy reasoned, "If I cause trouble, Daddy will spend even less time at home." Now as an adult she thinks similarly, "If I'm a trouble-maker, my husband will leave me just like Daddy left me." So she avoids dealing with issues that threaten her third failing marriage.

Nancy also concluded as a child that Daddy was absent because she was unworthy of his attention. If she were better, prettier, etc., he would have stayed home more. Nancy's father never told her these things and probably didn't believe them, but she inferred them from his actions.

Later in life Nancy learned a healing truth. Her father was absent because he had baggage of his own from his imperfect childhood. He felt that he was basically bad and unlovable. Therefore he worked his you-know-what off at the office to prove to his family and the world that he was a good enough provider.

Ironically Nancy's father loved his family. He just didn't know how to get past his own baggage to be able to love them the way they wanted to be loved—with his time and attention. He probably had a deep-down, unmet need to be affirmed since he never received that from his parents while growing up. So he tried to get it through the acquisition of money and power. He was just another hurt person who ended up hurting his kids. I guess that's why people say, "Hurt people hurt people."

I Thought I Was Enormous

On a recent trip home to visit my aging mother I decided to organize her huge collection of old photographs into an actual photo album. I liked the idea of putting the pictures in chronological order so I could see my family history in black and white.

As I put the pictures in order, I found photos of myself as a young child that I had never seen before. Seeing these pictures allowed me to see how my body changed as I grew up. It was an eye-opening experience.

Interestingly I remembered myself to be freakishly huge during my elementary school years. But in reality I wasn't the ponderous blimp that I remembered. It wasn't until my early teen years that I started putting on weight at a more alarming rate.

It's sad that I felt so bad about myself long before I actually gained the weight. It's almost as if I grew into obesity like it was a self-fulfilling prophecy. I saw myself as huge, so I eventually became huge.

Thankfully later in life God corrected my misperceptions in the light of His merciful truth. And He can and will do the same for you so you can see yourself and others through the eyes of love instead of through eyes of critical self-judgment and condemnation.

Kids Misunderstand Sometimes

Recently my teenagers told me something that really cracked me up. I was in the middle of explaining the content of this book to them—the part about how early childhood perceptions can be distorted. That's when they simultaneously had a "light bulb moment" and said, "Oh! You mean like in *Toy Story*?"

My daughter, Lindsey, went on, "I know it sounds funny, but I totally believed my toys came to life when I left my bedroom, just like in the *Toy Story* movie. I used to stand outside my bedroom with the door almost closed, spying through a crack in the door to see if I could catch the toys moving." My son, Cory, agreed, also laughing, "I totally did that too! I used to look at them out of the corner of my eye and just wait…"

Fortunately Cory's and Lindsey's childhood misperceptions were amusing and not harmful. But I can't say the same for all of those childhood misunderstandings. Some childhood misperceptions mess up kids later in life.

One of my patients is a first-generation Asian American, born to an immigrant mother, as I was. The whole time she was growing up, when she acted naughty, her mother told her, "Be heavy, be heavy!" After the "be heavy" it sounded like her mom said, "...in the heart." My poor patient grew up thinking she was supposed to be sullen and serious all the time—heavy in her heart. Can you see how that could lead to depression?

Fast-forward to about a year ago, and new light was shed on the situation. When my patient finally asked her mother, "Mom, why did you always tell me, 'Be heavy in your heart'? The mom said, "What are you talking about? I was telling you, 'Behave!'"

Still other types of childhood misperceptions leave even more damaging effects, such as the one that affected my patient Bob when he was a little boy.

Six-year-old Bobby suffered a double-whammy when he lost his daddy in a car wreck many years ago. In addition to being left without a father, Bobby concluded that the accident was his fault: "I killed Daddy because he was coming home from work to see me when he died. He always came home as fast as he could because he missed me."

If six-year-olds could reason as well as adults, Bobby wouldn't have grown up feeling so incredibly guilty. Moreover, he might not have stuffed himself with so many french fries to feel better starting a short time after his dad died. But six-year-olds see the world through six-year-old perceptions, and that means they process information less accurately than adults. Not that adults do better in many cases.

Adult Traumas

For the purposes of this book I focus on childhood traumas as they relate to the emotions that trigger you in the present day. However, I don't mean to discount the impact of traumas that occur during your adult life. Adult traumas absolutely cause stress and evoke fear, just as childhood traumas do. And they can certainly contribute to your reaching for false comforters.

Some adult events are so awful they would traumatize even people with minimal preexisting baggage. I've counseled survivors of rape, sexual abuse, military horror, witnessed suicide, the Oklahoma City bombing, losses of loved ones, accidents, natural disasters, and other traumatic events. They came to me because of physical pain, but I found that their pain stemmed from a mixture of physical, emotional, and spiritual causes.

However, the reason I focus on childhood experiences instead of adult traumas in this book is because childhood is when you're the most vulnerable. If your own divorce triggered the same sense of abandonment you felt when Daddy walked out on you and Mommy forty years ago, then I want to treat the young you that was abandoned by Daddy. Once I get that version of you feeling better, the adult you tends to feel better also.

Small Events Can Lead to Big Lies

Myrna is an elderly woman now, but back when she was a four-year-old, she came down with polio and had to be hospitalized for a year in an "iron lung," which was the old term for a ventilator. She nearly died.

While it's true that she had polio, part of her overall perception of the experience was false. As a child she believed that she contracted polio as a punishment from God because she stole a small toy from her neighbor's house. She never verbalized this belief, so no adult was able to correct her thinking. As a result, she carried this sense of guilt with her into adulthood. As an adult she knew intellectually that polio was due to a virus. But at the same time she believed on an emotional level that it was her fault.

Myrna's example shows that not all life-changing circumstances are severely traumatic. Perhaps you were not abused in any horrific way as a child. Maybe you think you had perfect parents and a storybook-perfect childhood. Maybe you're even right about that.

However, the kind of distorted beliefs I'm talking about can come about from things such as childhood trips to the emergency room for broken bones, cuts (with bleeding), falling off your bike, illnesses, being left with an unfamiliar babysitter (which can be scary, no matter how nice the sitter is), having to sleep in the dark when you're afraid, and other events that fall short of bona fide "abuse" or "neglect."

The reason you can be traumatized by seemingly small events is because you're a child when these events occurred. To understand how seemingly small things can cause fear or irrational beliefs in a child, you have to allow yourself to think (and feel) like a child for a while. You must allow yourself to see things through the eyes you had *back then*, not the eyes you see through now.

Time Doesn't Necessarily Heal

We may forget about past hurts on an intellectual level, but we don't necessarily forget emotionally. If anything we wall off those hurtful memories as if they're abscesses, as discussed by Pastor Quinn Schipper in his book *Trading Faces*.[1]

An abscess is basically a bag of pus that forms in the body around bacteria and foreign bodies such as splinters in order to protect the body from a more generalized infection. It's a way to keep the infection contained.

Repressed emotional trauma from past experiences is also like an abscess. We tend to wall off painful memories in our minds in the same way the body forms abscesses around bacteria because we don't want to think about them.

For an abscess to heal, it must be located, opened, and drained of the poison. If it's not located and drained, it can continue to make the person ill and even kill him or her. That's why we perform CT scans of people's bellies when they have an unexplained fever. We look for hidden abscesses that generate toxins that secretly poison the person from the inside out.

It can hurt momentarily when the doctor lances an abscess to drain it, and it can hurt momentarily when you have to revisit those past traumas on the way to your emotional healing. However, fear of momentary discomfort is not a wise reason to avoid proper treatment. It's like when you have a rotten tooth pulled. The discomfort lasts only for a very short time, but the relief you gain afterward is enormous and permanent.

If you feel uncomfortable about revisiting your childhood traumas, it's to be expected. Maybe that discomfort is a sign that you're on the right track.

Fear can be a major barrier to forgiveness. The fear of pain and discomfort that I note above are good examples. However, you might have other kinds of fear that block your forgiveness as well.

Perhaps you wonder, "Will I die or go off the deep end emotionally if I start thinking about what happened to me? What if I completely lose control and hurt myself or somebody else?" Or you might have an identity crisis: "What will be left of me once those bad feelings are gone? Who will I be? What will I think about if I no longer dwell on what he did to me?" Those questions can cause fear because any kind of change, even good change, can seem scary.

You Must Become Like a Little Child

Do you remember how much easier it was for you to forgive people when you were young? When somebody accidentally ran into you on the playground and then apologized, you rubbed your head for a minute, and then said, "That's OK." Instead of holding on to bitterness and resentment, you quickly forgave your classmate, shook off the hurt, and continued playing. You didn't hold grudges and continue to see the worst in people, as we learn to do later in life.

If you want to recover from whatever condition ails you, then pay attention because this is important. You must become like that adorable little child you once were. You must shed the restrictions the world has put on you—bitterness, negativity, envy—and instead put on compassion, mercy, and grace. That way you can more freely extend and receive healing forgiveness at a deep level and finally achieve radical well-being in mind, body, and spirit.

This book helps you do that in a way other books can't. It helps you to extend and receive forgiveness not only in your hardened adult mind but also in your innermost places, through the eyes of your softer, more teachable, inner child. Once your inner child goes through this process on an emotional level (and learns what God says about him or her—replacing the lies with truth, extending forgiveness, and receiving God's love), you experience deep healing, peace, and joy that nobody—not even the accuser—can ever steal away from you.

ACTION POINT
Questions to Ask God in Prayer

✿ Lord, will You search my innermost places for areas in which I need emotional, spiritual, and/or physical healing?

✿ If I need to revisit past memories, will You promise to help me do that at a rate I can handle?

✿ Lord, are there false beliefs mixed into my childhood memories? If so, please bring them to light. Are those beliefs about how I see myself? Or how I see You? Or someone else? Or some situation?

✿ Lord, in the place of those false beliefs, will You reveal healing truth? What is the truth about me, You, or the other person or situation?

Chapter 3

STRESS LESS, BETTY

URING HER SECOND visit with me, my five-foot-three, moderately overweight patient Betty announced, "Everything is fine, Doc! No emotional issues here!" But I had to wonder, "Does she truly believe her own words?"

As I reviewed Betty's intake paperwork from her initial visit, I saw red flags that indicated extreme stress. She was taking depression and anxiety medications and listed twenty-three drug allergies on her past medical history along with seven stress-induced illnesses: insomnia, unexplained hives, ulcers, migraines, unexplained hot flashes since age twenty-five, fibromyalgia, and irritable bowel syndrome.

Betty came to see me because of neck pain. Her X-rays and MRIs were normal, so on her very first visit I treated her with OMM and gave her soft tissue "trigger point" injections with numbing medicine. Even in the presence of stress, OMM and soft tissue injections usually help the patient at least a little. But in Betty's case, despite a 40 percent improvement in her pain at the end of her first visit, by the time she returned a week later she said she felt worse overall.

In addition to her ongoing pain in the days after I treated her, Betty continued to suffer from multiple drug allergies. Repressed stress seems to make certain bodies supersensitive to any kind of "invasion," even if it's invasion by injections or physical touch from a doctor. (When under stress people can even have unexplained, widespread hives, in addition to having a bazillion allergies. This is known as "stress urticaria.")

On top of her other issues I couldn't ignore Betty's weight problem. She said she gained seventy pounds in a short period of time in the few years before she came to me. You don't gain seventy pounds by accident. You gain that kind of weight when you eat for nonphysiological reasons such as stress, depression, and anxiety, or in response to some kind of major trauma.

When I looked at the whole picture—the negative imaging studies, the paradoxical worsening in response to OMM, her sudden weight gain, the bazillion allergies, and stress-induced illnesses—the real cause of her neck pain seemed obvious. Betty undoubtedly had emotional issues that she was medicating with food and carrying as physical pain.

Do you see how it works in medicine? In order to best diagnose and treat my patients, I have to do more than just listen to what they say. I also have to attune to them and understand who they are psychologically, emotionally, and even spiritually.

Before I go on, please let me clarify. I did not say that Betty's fibromyalgia, migraine pain, bowel dysfunction, and other illnesses were imaginary. I said only that stress makes physical, emotional, and pain problems worse in many cases. Stress may even initiate those illnesses before they take on a life of their own and cause secondary problems.

In addition I did *not* say that *all* patients with fibromyalgia, migraines, etc., have emotional or spiritual roots to their illnesses. In actual fact, only a subset of people with these conditions has emotional and/or spiritual roots to their illnesses. There are plenty of others with rheumatologic disorders such as lupus, rheumatoid arthritis, and the like who have fibromyalgia too, and theirs is unlikely to be substantially emotionally driven. That's not to say that stress doesn't make everybody's fibromyalgia symptoms worse, though!

As I said, your body deals with repressed emotional stress in a multitude of ways. When you bury your stress, the stress sometimes changes form and oozes out of your pores as physical pain, unwanted and unhealthy behaviors, and physical illness.

This mind-body-spirit connection is so powerful that my mentor, Dr. Stiles, emphasizes it repeatedly during his quarterly manual medicine weekend courses at Mercy Hospital in Oklahoma City. I know because I've attended at least twenty of these courses. At one of them in 2011 I personally heard Dr. Stiles say, "If people don't talk out their stress, their bodies will act out their stress."

Actually, at this particular class Dr. Stiles credited his pastor-friend Robert McAfee for the quotation, saying it was from one of their many private conversations. Don't you think it's interesting that both pastors and world-renowned, award-winning doctors came to the same conclusion? I do. The mind, body, and spirit are most definitely connected. Now let's go back to Betty's story to see how stress manifested physically in her case.

Betty's Next Visit

I had quite a challenge in front of me with Betty. I had to tell her that her complaints were emotionally driven. I had to motivate her to face whatever she was suppressing. I had to do all of this quickly and efficiently, as follow-up appointments supposedly last twenty minutes in my office. Yeah, right!

Because Betty didn't respond to my earlier, softer approach about the stress issue, I was more direct on her next visit. I'm not allowed to *slap* people because of that pesky "do no harm" oath. But I do know how to get their attention with my body language and tone of voice. That's where being an Italian from back East comes in handy. I am able to broadcast, "Snap out of it!" without actually saying it out loud.

I said, "Betty, let me review your intake paperwork. You reported having illnesses that are known to be stress-induced. You didn't check depression and anxiety off on our list, yet you take amitriptyline, which is an antidepressant, and you take alprazolam, which is an anxiety medicine. That tells me that you're in denial about your depression and anxiety. Plus you're allergic to twenty-three medicines, and you indicated that you recently experienced rapid weight gain, which means you've probably been eating for emotional reasons. Do you still think you aren't under stress?"

"That's not fair!" she said. "I don't take the anxiety medicine every day. I take it only as needed."

I replied, "What does that mean? Having anxiety every *other* day means you don't have anxiety?" I shouldn't have been sarcastic, but I guess the New York version of me showed up for work that day.

I saw Betty's jaw muscles tense up as she gritted her teeth, but she remained strikingly calm and even managed to smile. I suppose it comes from years of practice stuffing her emotions and denying her problems. "No, Doc. I told you I'm not stressed."

Since she wasn't open to talking about emotional issues, I told her I would not be able to manipulate her or give her more injections on the current visit. But the truth is I was testing her—was she really worse? If I helped her in some way that she didn't want to admit to herself, she'd protest. She'd want more of the treatment that, at first, she said didn't help.

I was right. Betty started back peddling as soon as I suggested we stop treatment. "Well, on second thought, maybe I'm a little better."

"Great! Because you're a little better, I'll let you go to PT two more times. That'll give you another week to pray and ask God if stress is part of your problem. If this doesn't work, maybe you and I can part ways for the time being. You can always come back in a few months or years if you remember some kind of emotional trauma that you think is related. Maybe you just need a little more time."

I went on to say, "By the way, I noticed a moment ago that you tensed up your jaws when we were talking about whether or not you have anxiety. I wonder if that means you 'grin and bear it' or try to 'swallow your stress' and 'gnash your teeth' rather than actually verbalize what's bothering you. Maybe you could chew on that between now and our next visit." Boy, oh boy, my approach paid off big time.

Allostasis and Heavy Emotional Loads

If my mentor, Dr. Stiles, treated Betty, he would have used the tension in her back as a gateway for dialoguing: "Betty, the tissues in your low back feel to me like they have a lot of tension on them. At any time in your life did you feel like something happened that caused you to pick up a heavy load, mentally or emotionally?" Or he might have said (while examining her back), "It feels to me like this tissue tension is somehow connected with a past traumatic event. Does any severely traumatic event come to mind as I touch this tense spot on your back?"

On the other hand, if Dr. Stiles were describing Betty to us doctors and therapists in a classroom-type setting, he would use medical terminology. He would say, "Betty has a high 'allostatic load.'" Dr. Stiles uses the term *allostasis* to describe the heightened state of stress that leads to deleterious physical changes of pain and illness. He credits Bruce McEwen, PhD, for having coined the term.[1]

When Dr. Stiles talks about allostasis in his manual medicine courses, he cites a research study that came out of San Francisco in 1992. In this study the people who had the worst outcomes after back surgery were those who had significant childhood trauma. Patients who had three or more out of five possible kinds of trauma had an 85 percent chance of having ongoing back pain after surgery, whereas patients who had no childhood trauma had only a 5 percent incidence of failure of their back surgery. This study shows how past emotional trauma can affect your current perception of pain.[2] As you will find out, Betty had a number of past traumas that were at play to affect her perception of pain through the phenomenon of allostasis.

The "Lies" Were Revealed

The night before Betty's last appointment with the physical therapist, her emotional dam broke. She was going to have to see me in a couple days, and she knew I would stop all treatment if she failed to improve. So, reluctantly, she faced her fears and prayerfully allowed some pretty bad memories to come to the surface.

When Betty was seventeen years old, her drug-addicted, physically abusive boyfriend told her if she left him, he would kill himself. Sure enough, after he threatened her with a baseball bat, she left him, and he ended his life via carbon monoxide poisoning.

In the here and now Betty lived with unfathomable fear that her husband would find out the truth about her old boyfriend's death. Deep down she believed the lie that he might abandon her just as the old boyfriend abandoned her by killing himself.

Part of her guilt was over the death of her boyfriend, and the other part was from keeping that story from her husband. The longer she kept the truth from him, the more shame she felt. And the more she feared his leaving her.

When the dam finally broke, Betty told her husband of many years about what happened with this old boyfriend. She tearfully begged for his forgiveness over having kept the secret from him. He gladly offered it and also told her, "It's OK, Honey. I still love you." Because her husband loved her, he had nothing but compassion for her.

To quote Dr. Stiles yet again, "It's not so much what happened to them but how they perceive it." Betty perceived this buried secret to be more dangerous than it actually was. Once she faced the truth, nothing bad happened.

It was like the fear of Y2K that some people had back in 1999. They stockpiled firewood and canned goods, expecting some kind of apocalypse, but when the year 2000 came, nothing bad happened. In the same way, once you find the right kind of help and face the traumatic or shameful things you've been suppressing, things will get better for you, not worse.

Things most definitely got better for Betty. Along with her emotional catharsis (the confession and subsequent crying) came a physical catharsis. The day after telling her husband that story, she had the biggest and best bowel movement of her lifetime. In "hind" sight (pun intended) Betty realized that her bowel problems were from stress.

After getting to know Betty further, we jokingly named this bowel movement "the dump of a lifetime." She felt like she eliminated a lifetime of waste that she held in.

It makes sense for a patient to have a huge bowel movement at the termination of stress. Stress causes the body to be in a fight-or-flight, high-adrenaline mode. When your body is under stress, it diverts blood away from the bowels and to the muscles so you can run away from the saber-tooth tiger. Once the threat of the tiger disappears, blood goes back to the intestines, and gastrointestinal function is finally allowed to proceed normally.

It's not like Betty is the only one who has experienced this phenomenon of improved bowel movements with reduction of stress. My physical therapist mentor, Micha Sale, PT, also talks about patients who have had "dumps of a lifetime" under her amazingly expert, Christ-centered manual medicine care.

Bye-bye, irritable bowel syndrome; hello, "dump of a lifetime." If you want normalized bowel function, don't succumb to the advertising messages from the "probiotic" yogurt companies. No matter what the Hollywood actress on the TV commercial tells you, stress reduction beats probiotic yogurt in regard to normalizing your bowel movements any day.

It Got Even Better

As you might expect, the release of pent-up stress caused Betty's ulcers and lower abdominal pain to totally disappear, and the OMM and injections began to work, her fibromyalgia pain lessened, and she experienced a substantial reduction in the frequency of her migraines. And all of this happened over only a few days' time.

Betty had some pretty amazing epiphanies from God during those first few weeks after her catharsis. On visit number three Betty told me that she realized why she gained the seventy pounds from stress eating. She also realized why she got so much worse pain-wise in the few years before she came to me: her last child (or should I say, her last "distraction"?) left home. Once she had an empty nest, she subconsciously created a new distraction: she ate and focused her mind on physical illness to avoid memories from her past that were even more painful.

Betty also stopped having hot flashes. She had been having them several times a week ever since her hysterectomy about twenty-five years before. However, within a few days of her catharsis they stopped completely. A few weeks later she had one "try" to come on, but she stopped it dead in its tracks by taking her thoughts captive and righting them. When she felt her left ear begin to get hot (that's how all her hot flashes started), she said, "No! I don't need to have hot flashes anymore!"

Did you catch that little nuance in Betty's word choice? When Betty relayed the story to me, I said, "*Hold it!* Did you hear what you said?" She paused for a minute and then had a huge "Aha!" moment. She said, "Yes! I don't *need* them anymore."

She understood what I meant immediately. Those hot flashes were something she needed at one time because they distracted her from feeling guilt over her ex-boyfriend's suicide. In a twisted way they helped her. They were her temporary solution. They were an unlikely "false comforter."

On that visit I reassured Betty that it was perfectly OK for her to need those medical problems as crutches for all those years. She wasn't bad for needing a crutch. She was wounded. Wounded people need crutches.

I wanted her to reject any guilt she might feel for having had stress-induced medical problems, because that too could have been fodder for a new attack from the accuser. "You're bad because you had stress-induced medical problems."

Ha ha! Praise God for my ability to stay one step ahead of that little, lying jerk. (I mean the accuser, not Betty).

Betty's Long-Term Outcome

I've known Betty for about four years. During that time she's maintained about an 80 percent to 90 percent reduction of all of her stress-induced physical problems. Part of her success is due to godlier thinking, and another part is due to my treatment. However, some of Betty's relief came from her finding healthier ways to deal with stress.

Betty still has recurrences of pain about twice a year though. When Betty has a recurrence of neck pain and tells me, "No, I didn't have trauma. I didn't fall, I didn't have a car wreck, and I didn't lift anything heavy. I just woke up with the pain," I know that something is up emotionally. Maybe a new layer of old, repressed lies or fears?

At those times I manipulate her body and inject her tight muscles to relieve the pain, but I also help her take her emotions captive. Instead of letting her dwell on the pain, I get her to ask herself, "What emotion do I feel right now?" Simply by identifying the emotion, she sometimes experiences less pain automatically.

In an unexpected way Betty has even become grateful to God for her physical pain. It's her way of recognizing that she's bottling up her emotions. It's like her emotional litmus test for stress.

ACTION POINT
Questions to Ask God in Prayer

✿ Lord, will You reveal the true sources of the stress in my life? Is it something other than what I dwell on at the surface level?

✿ If I can't hear Your answer, is it because I am up against a barrier I created to protect myself?

✿ Is it safe to get past this barrier?

✿ What is the cause of the barrier? Do I believe a lie about myself, You, others, a situation, or an event from the past? Or are sin or unforgiveness blocking me from getting through? If I still feel blocked, will You help me overcome my barrier and show me truth, anyway?

PART TWO

THE WHOLE YOU
Connecting Mind, Body, and Spirit

Chapter 4

A WHOLE IN THREE

MY PATIENT ALAN had a fully herniated disk in his low back. In order to avoid back surgery, he needed to follow my instructions to a tee. That meant he needed to have spinal cortisone shots, physical therapy, and lifting restrictions at work.

But at first Alan did the opposite of what I suggested. Rather than take time off from work and attend physical therapy, he voluntarily took on extra responsibilities at the office. He said he needed to cover for his coworker, Vince, whose wife was sick with breast cancer. He wanted to let Vince help her recover after a mastectomy.

I frequently hear about patients' work-related stress. They think that work is actually their main source of stress—even more than family relations. I think some of those people are wrong. Many people have deeper, lie-based childhood triggers that are set off by but not caused by their work environments.

It feels safer to think, "My work stresses me out," rather than, "Ever since my childhood, I've felt stupid, worthless, and incapable, and now I'm worried my superiors at work will figure out what an idiot I am and fire me." Alan definitely believed deep-seated lies about himself that worsened his back problems. Work was definitely contributing, but it took me a while to get the big picture.

Alan is one of those people who would give you the shirt off his back. Vince, the coworker who implored Alan to cover for him, is a liar who would take it. I can say this because they're both my patients, and I know them well. Vince has gambling problems, and when he falls into gambling binges, he lies to and takes advantage of everyone around him, including his coworker Alan.

Eventually, through prayer and dialoguing, Alan received truth from God about this situation. Previously Alan believed that his well-being was not as important as others' and that he didn't "deserve" to take time to care for himself. That's why he volunteered to help Vince when he should have let one of the younger, healthier guys at work cover for him.

If you don't deal with your deep-down lies, they deal with you. Stress can literally create illness and pain. Moreover, the lies associated with your stress can lead you to make bad choices that further compromise your health. For example, the "I'm not as valuable as other people" lie led Alan pretty close to needing back surgery.

In this chapter I explain the mind-body-spirit connection in greater detail so you can better understand how stress can become physical. I also tell you about the most mind-bending case of stress-induced illness that I have seen in my eighteen years of being a doctor.

Stabbed in the Back

When Alan finally got with the program, I treated him with pills, physical therapy, and epidural steroid injections to reduce the inflammation around that bad disk. About a month later, after his disk cooled off, I started using OMM on him to correct the body-wide alignment problems that caused wear and tear on that disk in the first place.

The third OMM treatment is when everything fell into place (and I don't just mean his spinal alignment). That was when I noticed a very tight spot at the midpoint of Alan's left shoulder blade. It radiated from between his shoulder blades straight through to the front of his chest. It literally felt like a hard foreign body was in there. I took this as an opportunity to get symbolic and ask some open-ended questions. Even if I'm off base with my questions, it doesn't really matter. As long as I get patients talking *somehow*, they eventually stumble onto the emotional aspects of their pain.

After feeling around on his back a little longer, I said, "Alan, I know your low back hurts, but when I touch higher, between your shoulder blades, it feels like there's a tightness that radiates straight through to the front of your chest and is limiting your breathing. By chance, did something break your heart...or take your breath away? Or might you be 'holding your breath,' worried about something bad that might happen? Or is there something you need to get off your chest?"

"Yeah, Doc, I know exactly what that means. There's a knife stuck in there. One of the guys at work really took advantage of me, and I'm still pretty mad about it. He borrowed money from me, supposedly to help pay for his wife's mastectomy, but it turns out she wasn't even sick. He just took that money and blew it at the casino. He just got fired over it because somebody saw him at the casino on his so-called sick days."

Even though I figured Alan was talking about my other patient, Vince, I couldn't admit it because of confidentiality laws. I also couldn't let on that I wondered if Alan was more hurt than angry. Men like to call negative emotions "anger" because anger feels manly and powerful, but oftentimes they just feel hurt, ashamed, belittled, or betrayed.

As Alan continued to unload about the situation, and as I continued to work on his back and chest, he loosened up very quickly. He even felt and heard a few pops in his back, indicating that his release of soft tissue tension was allowing his spinal alignment to return to normal.

It only made sense. At first when Alan's soft tissues were tense because of his pent-up bitterness, it was like I was playing tug-of-war with his muscles during OMM. But when he "let go" of the emotional tension, he also let go of the physical tension. In turn that allowed him to experience more substantial and permanent relief through the treatment.

Stress, Bad Health Habits, and Insomnia

Even before his back injury Alan suffered with insomnia, and it got worse after his injury. Part of the problem was the stress of being off work and lying in bed with racing thoughts, wondering what the injury meant for his future. Another part of it was the pain medicine. Usually hydrocodone mellows people out. But sometimes it winds them up and makes them hyper, as it did with Alan.

I did what I could to help him by changing his medicine. However, by far the best thing I did, in hindsight, was address his other health habits that could have been affecting his sleep. We call this "sleep hygiene."

First, I addressed his consumption of caffeine and sugar and his use of tobacco. Think about how these substances affect the physical body and, in turn, our emotions. Overconsuming caffeine not only makes people irritable, but it also impairs their sleep and makes them grouchy. In turn, having impaired sleep can contribute to a body-wide pain condition called fibromyalgia.

Nicotine can do the same. It's a stimulant just like caffeine. But it also causes cancer and kills you. That's how my own father died. He smoked two packs of filterless Camels a day for more than fifty years, and the cancer finally caught up with him when he was in his early seventies. He developed small-cell lung carcinoma and died seven weeks and two days after he was diagnosed.

Now let's talk about sugar. It tastes good going down, but after your blood sugar level drops, you crash and feel horrible. I wish I could say I learned my lesson over the years, but I haven't. I still love sweets, and I still eat them in abundance. I just can't eat them too late at night or I lie in bed with racing thoughts. (As you can see, I have the confession part down. It's just the repentance part that I'm having trouble with in this area.)

In addition to sugar, it's possible that other foods contribute to alterations in mood and even, indirectly, our ability to sleep at night. Though we don't know exactly how to connect the dots and explain why that happens, some have theorized that the neurotransmitter serotonin is involved. Interestingly serotonin is also one of the chemicals involved in sleep!

Getting back to Alan, to address his insomnia I got him to switch to drinking decaffeinated coffee and soda throughout the day, as well as promise to not eat sweets or smoke cigarettes in that four-hour window before bedtime. Not only did he normally smoke before bedtime, but he had also been in the habit of eating a Snickers bar, and chocolate contains both caffeine and sugar, which, as I said, are stimulants.

There's one more thing. Even though it's not ideal, I had him only "cut down" on his smoking rather than quit altogether. The reason I didn't have him quit entirely is that the poor guy was already going through a lot. Making him quit completely would have been too traumatic at that point.

Just making these modest changes helped him noticeably in terms of his sleep. And as a side benefit, because we took away many of his chemical stimulants, Alan's nighttime "restless leg syndrome" got better too. That's a condition where you can't help but move your legs at night because you're so uncomfortable.

Seeing the improvement in his sleep pattern after making only small changes, Alan, on his own, quit smoking completely and now limits his caffeine intake to only one caffeinated beverage each morning. He still eats his Snickers bar as well, but he eats it earlier in the day around lunchtime. By bedtime the effects of the daytime sugar and caffeine are long gone. Between those dietary and lifestyle changes and the exercise I have him do first thing in the morning, he now sleeps much better at night—*without medication.*

Biblical Proof of the Mind-Body-Spirit Connection

First Thessalonians 5:23 says, "And the very God of peace sanctify you wholly; and I pray God your whole spirit and soul and body be preserved blameless unto the coming of our Lord Jesus Christ" (KJV). Did you catch the parts in this scripture about the "spirit and soul and body" and about being sanctified "wholly"? For total health and wholeness you need to think about how those three dimensions affect each other.

The Bible is clear about how emotions affect the physical body. On two occasions Job said fear caused his bones to shake (Job 4:14–15). And according to Proverbs 14:30, "A calm and undisturbed mind and heart are the life and health of the body, but envy, jealousy, and wrath are like the rottenness of the bones" (AMP).

As if that isn't proof enough, in Luke 21:26 Jesus talked about "men's hearts failing them for fear, and for looking after those things which are coming on the earth: for the powers of heaven shall be shaken" (KJV).

Oddly, when I read about "men's hearts failing them for fear," I can't help but think about a very weird stress-induced heart condition known as Takotsubo cardiomyopathy. That's when sudden, very extreme stress leads to heart failure, arrhythmias, and death. It can even lead to actual rupture of the heart muscle due to sudden stress-induced changes in blood pressure. Because of stress men's hearts really can "fail them for fear." I don't *need* science to support that God's Word is true, but I like when it does.

How Emotions Become Physical

Another patient's story perfectly illustrates how subconscious emotions become physical. When I first met Anna, I didn't know about her past. I knew only that when I touched her pale, cold, and clammy back to examine her, she tensed up and shrugged her shoulders upward and forward, as though she was trying to protect herself or pull away from my touch.

Subconsciously shrugging her shoulders all the time is part of the reason Anna had neck pain and shoulder pain. This posture stresses the muscles and tends to pull the bones out of their correct alignment, further adding to muscle spasms and knots in the muscles. It's a vicious cycle.

I know about this postural response to stress from my own life too. As I sat in the dentist's chair during my recent root canal, I became aware of the fact that I was shrugging my shoulders in fear. Once I noticed my posture, I chose to let go of the mental tension (aka fear) and intentionally will my mind to relax. As soon as I did that, my shoulders fell back into a relaxed state and the tightness in my middle back went away.

Anna also had back and leg pain. However, an exhaustive search for the cause of Anna's back and leg symptoms revealed nothing. All of the imaging was negative. Her physical exam was negative. Based on all the available medical evidence, and despite her perception of back pain, she did not actually have an identifiable back problem.

Almost at the last minute before telling her, "I don't know...maybe I can't help," I noticed the extremely tense posture with which she sat on the exam table. Instead of allowing her legs to dangle loosely off the side of the table, she held her thighs together very tightly, as if she was trying subconsciously to keep somebody from prying them apart. At the same time her facial expression revealed no awareness of what her legs were doing.

Seeing the extreme tension in her thighs (and her lack of awareness of this tension), I asked her if she had been sexually abused in the past. Sure enough, between the ages of five and twelve years, Anna was sexually abused by her stepfather. It would have gone on longer, except daddy dearest went to jail on drug charges.

Being sure to get Anna's permission (for obvious reasons), and knowing how much strain must have been in her thigh muscles, I looked for "trigger points" or knots in the muscles of the upper inner thighs. Those are the muscles she used to squeeze her knees together, and trigger points in those muscles can cause numbness and tingling all the way to the inner ankle area.

I injected the knots (again, with her permission because the last thing I wanted to do was cause her to feel "violated" yet again), and by the grace of God she felt about 80 percent better. Nothing else had helped her that much, ever.

The take-home message is that emotions literally cause physical tension in your body, often through your assuming subconscious, protective postures. That means you must pay attention not only to your emotions but also to the posture caused by your emotions.

The Most Interesting Case

I finished my medical training about fourteen years ago, but every now and then I think about one of my patients from back when I was in residency. Her case was the most fascinating of my entire residency from a psychological point of view.

Cynthia was a forty-five-year-old physical therapy assistant with high blood pressure. Her children brought her to the hospital because she began to experience weakness on her left side and slurring of her speech. They figured she'd had a stroke. On admission Cynthia was completely paralyzed on one side and had slurred speech, just as you'd expect in someone who'd had a stroke.

But a full neurologic workup was negative. The head CT showed no bleeding. The MRI of her brain showed no clot. The blood work and spinal tap showed no infection or meningitis. She didn't have a stroke, she didn't have an inflammatory blood vessel condition, and she didn't have a nerve disease.

She wasn't lying, either. It turned out she had a real medical diagnosis that justified a stay in the rehab unit where I worked—but it was a psychological, not physical, diagnosis. She had what was called a conversion disorder. It was a psychosomatic reaction created by her mind in response to an intense emotional stress that she couldn't handle. The conversion took her mind off the stress. The physical symptoms were easier to wrap her mind around than was the emotional event that drove her over the edge.

Though conversion disorders are fairly uncommon (I've see only two in fourteen years of seeing pain-management patients), they happen frequently enough to be worth mentioning. Cynthia's case is a great and rather extreme example of how stress becomes physical.

At the time of Cynthia's admission to our rehab unit, the lead doctor put me in charge of the intake meeting with Cynthia's family. In that meeting the nurses, therapists, social workers, and psychologists were to give their initial reports, and I was to explain Cynthia's diagnosis, treatment plan, and prognosis to her family. Yet I barely understood her diagnosis myself! I knew only a tiny bit about it from my psychiatry rotation in medical school.

The lead doctor gave me succinct thirty-second blurb on how to handle the meeting. She said, "Patients with conversion disorders are highly amenable to the power of suggestion. If you convince her that the symptoms will pass, they will. So tell her you know exactly what's wrong with her, that it's treatable, and that it should take her exactly four days to get over it, because that's the amount of time we'll be paid by the insurance company to keep her on the unit."

Great. I felt like I was being thrown to the wolves. I thought I was training to be a doctor, not an actress.

As I walked in to the family meeting, I had an epiphany regarding how I could handle this meeting. I said, "As you know, this is the decade of the brain." (Meanwhile I was thinking, "I have no clue if this is still the decade of the brain.")

I went on to say, "After all the research that's been done, we understand only 10 percent of how the brain works. Clearly the brain functions in ways that we don't fully understand. The imaging studies are negative. Yet look at Cynthia. She's paralyzed—for the moment, anyway."

I had a captive audience. They were hanging on my every word. Even I believed what I was saying (sort of).

I went on to say, "There must be some neural connections that we don't totally understand that create strokelike symptoms in the absence of actual structural defects. The great news is when we *don't* see abnormalities on the tests, the symptoms resolve quickly. By Thursday she should be able to walk and use her arm totally normally. She'll need physical and occupational therapy while she's on our unit, and she will need emotional counseling to deal with the stress that's associated with these recent events. But other than that, there's nothing else to do. And just in case you're wondering, this will never recur."

I couldn't have handled it more perfectly. Everything I said was true (in a way). The patient progressed dramatically fast, *much* faster than an actual stroke patient could ever progress. It took her four days to make more progress than the average stroke patient makes in a lifetime.

Unfortunately there was one area that I forgot to address in the family meeting. I forgot to address her speech disorder. Her arm and leg were working much better, but her speech was just as bad as it was on the day of admission.

The speech pathologist on the unit caught up with me on the third day of the patient's stay and told me the bad news about my oversight.

Fortunately I was able to see the patient on the same day and convince her that her speech problem would resolve by the end of that day (which it did, thanks be to God).

As I got to know this patient, I deduced the cause of her underlying stress. Her fiancé left her for another woman three days before the onset of her illness. This abandonment caused her to feel helpless, alone, and frightened, just like many of the elderly stroke patients she worked with in her job as a physical therapy assistant.

Because of Cynthia's prior experience with stroke patients, her subconscious mind knew how to mimic a stroke when faced with the stressor. So Cynthia just shut down with paralysis rather than break down emotionally.

The Pressure Cooker Analogy

I think we hold on to stress as though we're pressure cookers. When the heat goes up, we get hot inside. But from the outside you can't tell at first. After a certain point when the pressure goes up to a threshold level, a little steam comes out. That pressure release keeps the pressure cooker from exploding.

In a way those mysterious pain recurrences that you just wake up with out of the blue can be like your pressure cooker letting off just enough steam to keep you from exploding. Any time a patient says, "I just woke up with it hurting," I entertain the possibility of stress (immediately after ruling out the more dangerous diagnoses, of course).

If your weakness is not physical pain, your pressure release could come in the form of an alcoholic, food, shopping, or gambling binge; insomnia; excessive sleeping; hoarding; cutting; pulling out your hair (it's called trichotillomania); a trip to the casino; cutting or picking at yourself; and various other compulsions too numerous to mention. Those things are really all the same. They're just different manifestations of stress.

By the same token your stress may come in other physical manifestations that I didn't mention. Your ulcer may flare, your blood pressure may go up, you might get a bout of migraine headaches or a flare in your muscles, or you might have seizures, restless legs, sleepwalking, or facial tics. You could also have an outbreak of shingles or other rashes or infections.

Another one of my patients has been to a half-dozen dermatologists, and none of them have figured out the source of her rashes. Hello, people! It's stress! Why are other doctors so afraid to say that? What are the chances that every single dermatologist she visited was an idiot? Pretty slim. If you've seen a lot of doctors and nobody knows what's wrong with you, maybe it's stress.

Do yourself a favor. If your pain level, overeating, or physical illness increases abruptly, stop and ask yourself, "What's going on at work or at home right now? How do I feel emotionally? What have I been thinking about?" Identifying the real issue is the first step toward finding lasting peace.

Nothing to "Blow Off"

Some stress-induced pains can be dangerous, so don't blow them off. It's tempting to say, "This is no big deal. It's only stress-induced." But that doesn't mean the stress won't kill you!

When Betty experienced chest pain last year, she called me before she contacted her internist. She had a fight with her husband the night before she called our office, so she figured her chest pain was stress-induced. She thought, "It's no big deal."

Wrong. Betty was on the edge of a heart attack. Thank goodness she called me. We were able to get her internist involved before anything bad happened. She had an 80 percent blockage of her left anterior descending coronary artery and was probably a few weeks away from having the kind of heart attack known as a "widow-maker." Thank God for cardiologists, stents, medicines, technology, and discernment!

As I said, stress contributes to physical disease, but then the physical disease can take on a life of its own. That's why it helps to have a doctor who really knows you.

God gave us doctors, medicines, and procedures for a reason—to be used wisely. Be wise, like Betty. Report your symptoms to your doctor and let him or her run the necessary tests. If the tests come back negative for physical illness, you can ask yourself, "Could this be emotional?" after the dust settles.

In the next chapter I introduce you to numerous other medical conditions that can be, and frequently are, caused by or contributed to by stress.

ACTION POINT
Questions to Ask God in Prayer

✡ Lord, are my physical pains and symptoms in any way caused or amplified by emotional or spiritual stress?

✡ Will You help me identify what past events or relationships, if any, are involved?

✡ Will You provide me with better ways to release my emotional and/or spiritual burdens than through my physical body?

✡ If I'm having trouble hearing You, will You please come to my side of the barrier and reveal truth to me anyway? Or help me get to Your side of the barrier somehow?

Chapter 5

NEW HOPE FOR PAIN SUFFERERS

THE MOMENT KEITH was served with divorce papers, he said it felt as if a vice grip attached itself to that big bump at the base of his neck. We doctors call that bump "vertebra prominens" because it's the most prominent bump in your lower neck. Some people call it the "buffalo hump."

With each line he read, he said it felt as if the grip tightened another notch. His wife wanted everything—the kids, the house, the car, the savings account, and the family business.

By the time he got to the end of the divorce papers, he was flared up in all of his usual pain areas. Yet he remained emotionally composed.

Maybe shock explained his superhuman degree of composure. But I think he just couldn't handle the emotions, so he subconsciously transformed his conflict into physical pain. It felt less threatening, I guess.

Different people express their emotional conflicts in different ways. Some remain emotionally collected (on the surface) but subconsciously transform their stress into rashes or digestive trouble. Others go on drinking, eating, drug, shopping, or gambling binges. Or they have flare-ups of their psychological disorders and lapse into depression or panic attacks.

In this chapter I build on what I told you in the last chapter by explaining the biological mechanisms for how stress becomes physical. I talk about the neural circuitry in your brain and how your posture changes during times of stress.

But even more important I tell you about two commonly missed physical diagnoses that could be adding to your pain. Partly because of the posture people adopt while under stress (and after trauma), many individuals develop soft tissue problems that doctors often fail to recognize. In this chapter I distinguish these conditions from a different medical problem called fibromyalgia. And I explain how to find practitioners in your geographical area who can properly diagnose and treat these often-missed conditions.

Some of the information in this chapter is a bit complex, but the take-home message is simple. By addressing both the emotional and physical aspects of your pain, you can feel a whole lot better than you do right now.

It's Biological

For a minute let me talk about the neuronal circuits in your brain that govern emotions and physical pain. Don't worry if it sounds technical for a couple paragraphs. I get to the easy-to-understand point pretty quickly.

Certain more primitive parts of your brain are involved in the processing of emotions. These areas include the limbic system, which houses the amygdala, as well as parts of the cerebral cortex called the limbic forebrain, anterior cingulate gyrus, and insular cortex.

In the more sophisticated frontal lobe, or cerebral area, the anterior cingulate gyrus allows you to focus attention on the source of your pain. So if the steam in a pot of boiling water just burned you, your anterior cingulate gyrus would increase your level of attention so you wouldn't get hurt worse.

The control of pain transmission (i.e., nerve endings complaining to your brain about the steam burn) occurs in a different area. Pain transmission from your injured nerve endings travels up to the brain and lands on the periaqueductal gray matter (PAG) in the midbrain and the rostral ventral nucleus (RVM) of the medulla. The PAG and RVM are relatively far from the emotions/attention parts of your brain. But interestingly there's a very strong nerve tract connection between those different areas of the brain. It's like when two rural towns that are geographically far from each other are connected by a stretch of highway.

If emotions didn't modulate your perception of pain, there would be no need for a biological connection between the two areas of your brain. You wouldn't need to connect two towns with an excellent, expensive stretch of highway if strong interaction didn't occur between those two towns.

The emotional parts of your brain actually talk to the pain-sensing parts of your brain through this communications highway, and they either calm you down to make the pain seem less intense or hype you up and make the pain seem worse. All this is done through the action of neurotransmitters, which include chemicals such as GABA (gamma-aminobutyric acid).

Let me point out that the primitive emotion part (amygdala) is also anatomically close to the part of your brain involved in memories (the hippocampus). They are close because, in reality, your memories and your emotions are biologically intertwined and work *together* to modulate your response to current physical pain. Memories of past, painful experiences affect how you perceive new pain experiences through a different stretch of the emotions-pain communications highway.

Assuming that I haven't lost you, let me explain why this emotions-pain connection is good news. It's proof that gaining control of your thoughts and emotions can actually modulate your perception of pain. The calmer and more peaceful you are when the pain occurs, the less it bothers you. It's also why hypnosis, biofeedback, and relaxation techniques work to help you feel less physical pain.

As if that's not cool enough, your more relaxed and healthier thinking can actually *change the function of your nerve cells* (at least to an extent) through a process called neuroplasticity. In other words, your brain is more like Play-Doh than it is like concrete. Its output can be changed for the better—no matter how old you are.

This doesn't mean patients whose pain is rooted in their emotions should leave their doctors' offices and find a good psychologist instead. Psychological counseling alone often isn't enough to heal their pain. My mentor, Dr. Ed Stiles, has a belief that I think will make a lot of sense when you consider the anatomy I just described. He once said (and I paraphrase), "Psychologists tend to help patients understand the source of their conflicts, but they may, in some cases, underestimate the power of tapping into the emotional element, where you get the actual resolution of conflicts."[1]

In the same OMM course Dr. Stiles went on to say, "There are two ways to tap into the real source of your patients' pain. One is through the musculoskeletal system, and the other is by accessing the emotions that are associated with their pain."[2] His hypothesis makes perfect sense based on how the brain is wired, and it probably explains why his methods allow us (his students) to deliver results so quickly.

It's not that psychologists can't tap into the emotional triggers causing their patients pain; it's just that they aren't allowed to physically touch their patients while talking with them. But an MD or DO can, and that allows us doctors who engage in OMM to get deeper into the patients' problems—and to get there faster too.

Stressful Postures and Pain

When we feel unpleasant emotions, our bodies automatically adopt certain postures. For instance, when afraid some people curl their shoulders forward and hang their heads down as if they're getting ready for a beating. They do this without even realizing it. I guess it's a form of self-protection.

The problem is, our poor muscles have to work hard to maintain these protective postures. It's no wonder they hurt. Subconsciously tensing muscles up all day long causes them to develop knots ("trigger points"). It also causes them to pull certain bones out of alignment, which in turn creates more pain. Keith did something like that, in that he hunched his shoulders when he read through the divorce papers. He hunched so hard that he made his whole body hurt.

If you think you might respond to stress the way Keith does, check the position of your shoulders right now (since I read your mind and made you nervous). Are they up next to your ear lobes? Or are they much lower, where they're supposed to be? If your shoulders are tense, let them relax. For some people it's harder to do than you might think. Practice doing this each time you catch yourself hunching up your shoulders when you're nervous, and soon your neck, shoulders, and back may hurt less.

Physical Reactions to Emotional Stress

Did you know that stress can affect the function of your nerves? It does this by causing you to hyperventilate (take rapid, shallow breaths) and exhale more carbon dioxide than usual. In turn, the reduced level of CO_2 in your bloodstream affects the acid-base level of your blood. Since the acid-base level of your blood affects the conduction of electricity in your nerves, you end up feeling numbness and tingling around your mouth and in your fingers and toes!

Likewise, stress can lead you to grit or grind your teeth at night, which then causes temporomandibular joint (jaw) or tooth pain. Sometimes I see this in people who "grin and bear it" (i.e., swallow their emotions) or "bite their tongues" rather than confront situations that need to be corrected.

Stress can even aggravate soft tissue conditions such as fibromyalgia (where your whole body is tender to the touch). It can also lead to gastrointestinal conditions such as ulcers (where you have abdominal pain that is relieved by eating), nausea, vomiting, diarrhea, and irritable bowel syndrome (where eating causes abdominal pain and having bowel movements relieves it), and pelvic pain from interstitial cystitis (a condition in which bladder filling causes pain and emptying relieves it).

Let's not forget stress-induced immune disorders such as shingles (a painful, burning, and itchy rash due to the chicken pox virus); profound allergies (getting every side effect known to man each time a doctor gives you a new medicine); food and medicine intolerance; or unexplained rashes, acne, yeast infections, cold sores, staph outbreaks, or hives.

As if those symptoms aren't bad enough, forget about getting a good night's sleep when you're under stress. Many people suffer with stress-induced nightmares, insomnia, sleepwalking, or restless leg syndrome (where you feel creepy-crawly sensations in your legs at night and have to move them).

Psychological Reactions to Emotional Stress

There is a long list of psychiatric conditions that are worsened by stress, including but not limited to depression, anxiety, neurosis, psychosis, panic disorders, personality disorders, eating disorders, addictions, and "somatoform" disorders (where your subconscious stress comes out as physical symptoms). Usually pain is a prominent feature of somatoform disorders. Examples of somatoform disorders include conversion disorder, such as Cynthia's case in the previous chapter; hypochondriasis, a persistent preoccupation with the belief that your physical symptoms represent illness; and somatization disorder, where your stress turns into not just one but also a multitude of physical complaints.

All of these conditions are motivated by the person's need to assume the "sick" role. If a person has a somatoform disorder, he or she is *not* faking the symptoms or lying. The symptoms are very real and come about due to psychological/emotional factors.

Two Commonly Missed Sources of Pain

Of the patients who end up on my doorstep, many have seen other doctors and have been through every test known to man but still have been offered no clear explanation for why they hurt. And there's a good reason for this: not all pain-producing conditions can be verified with imaging where the doctor uses studies and lab work! Sometimes it takes an ultraspecialized kind of physical exam, using nothing but his or her hands for diagnosis.

I'm thinking in particular of two diagnoses that I see nearly every day in my pain-management practice. They are called myofascial pain syndrome (MPS) and somatic dysfunction (SD). In my experience many patients who have been told, "There's nothing wrong with you" or, "It's all in your head," by their other doctors (because their lab tests results were normal) actually have one or the other or both of these conditions!

On the upside neither MPS nor SD is dangerous, and their treatment is noninvasive, nonnarcotic, and inexpensive, especially compared to surgery. But on the downside patients might have to drive a long way to find the right kind of doctor, especially in the case of somatic dysfunction. Doctors who know how to recognize and treat these conditions well are few and far between. In the remainder of this chapter I tell you more about myofascial pain syndrome and somatic dysfunction, including how to find a doctor to screen you for them.

Myofascial Pain Syndrome

To be fair, most doctors in my specialty (physical medicine and rehabilitation, or "PM&R") know how to evaluate patients for MPS. But some of my colleagues in other specialties (anesthesiology-pain management, rheumatology, orthopedics, neurosurgery, etc.) might not be as likely to look for it.

We can't all be experts at everything! I don't know how to clip your brain aneurysm, replace your arthritic hip, treat your lupus, or put you to sleep for surgery *and wake you up afterward* (that's the tricky part). In the same way my colleagues in other specialties might not necessarily have had extensive training in regard to MPS.

With that being said, only a small number of us physiatrists (PM&R doctors) actually have a passion for treating MPS. So there's a chance that even if someone has seen a physiatrist, the MPS diagnosis still could have been missed.

If you have MPS, you are likely to experience numbness, tingling, and pain in your trunk or limbs. You may also have marble-sized knots in your muscles on physical examination. The knots may be small, but when compressed they can actually send numbness, tingling, and pain to distant areas, sometimes even into the arms and legs. We call this "referred pain."

Because of the numbness and tingling it can cause in the limbs, MPS is often misdiagnosed as pinched nerves in the spine. As such, patients are sent for MRIs and electrodiagnostic studies (EMGs) that don't end up revealing the real problem. Or worse, these tests show unrelated problems that, in turn, send doctors down the wrong paths.

The way to diagnose MPS is via a hands-on physical exam in which a specialist actually pokes all over the patient's body, looking for the knots. Basically the doctor's hands *are* the diagnostic test.

MPS has a very interesting history. It was first introduced broadly as a diagnosis in 1983 when Dr. Janet Travell, the former White House physician for Presidents John F. Kennedy and Lyndon Johnson, released her landmark book on the subject.

We now know President Kennedy had significant back problems, so it makes sense that he would recruit a doctor such as Janet Travell to the White House. She pioneered techniques to inject knotted muscles with nonnarcotic numbing medicine ("trigger point injections") to ease the pain, as well as the use of a physical therapy procedure called "spray and stretch." One could easily speculate that President Kennedy himself received this type of nonnarcotic pain treatment.

Interestingly my mentor, Dr. Stiles, a pioneer in the field of OMM, had dinner with Dr. Travell about twenty or twenty-five years ago after one of the last meetings of the North American Academy of Manual Medicine (NAAMM). He said Dr. Travell was quite elderly and confined to a wheelchair at the time.

During a break at this high-powered NAAMM conference, Dr. Stiles gave an impromptu talk about his concept of "sequencing." As he spoke to this group, which included Dr. Travell, he explained that "sequencing" in OMM involves screening the patient's entire body, looking for the most restricted area. Then that area is treated first, regardless of the location of the patient's symptoms. Afterward the patient is rescreened, with the specialist looking for the next tightest area, which would be treated second.[3]

According to his paradigm, the physiatrist just keeps repeating the process (screen, treat, screen, treat...), as if peeling the layers off an onion. Sometimes a distant body part (such as the foot and ankle or even the wrist or elbow) has to be treated to take pressure off of the body part that hurts. Otherwise the pain tends to come right back.

At the post-conference dinner later that day, Dr. Travell told Dr. Stiles she had an epiphany after hearing his impromptu speech that afternoon. She realized that throughout her career, she had sequenced her trigger point injections just as he sequenced his OMM! I would have loved to have been a fly on the wall listening in on that landmark conversation directly.

Based on what I have seen in my own pain-management practice, sequencing does seem to yield superior and longer-lasting results, just as these two icons (Drs. Travell and Stiles) have pointed out. Using the language in my field, one might say, "Properly sequenced treatment gets into the patient's deeper layers faster." Thus it would be optimal for your doctor to be familiar with this approach and also use it regularly. To find a doctor who can evaluate you for MPS, visit the American Academy of Physical Medicine and Rehabilitation's website at www.aapmr.org and click on the link to find a physiatrist in your area.

Somatic Dysfunction

The other commonly missed diagnosis I want to tell you about is somatic dysfunction (SD). Often SD runs hand in hand with MPS. Patients who have one diagnosis tend to have the other.

Often the pain of SD "bounces around" from one body part to another. One day the patient might feel neck pain, and the next day his neck might feel fine but his tailbone might hurt. That's because as bones, muscles, and joints shift in the body to compensate for the cause of the pain, physical forces and tension in the body shift as well.

A very common area of pain in SD is the sacroiliac joints (SI joints), which are at those dimples next to the spine in the low back/upper buttock area. Lots of times the underlying problem causing the SI joint pain isn't even at the joint itself. More often than not the underlying problem that causes SI joint pain is higher up in the middle back, and the SI joints are hurting because they're compensating.

Other areas that may hurt in SD include the area between or next to the shoulder blades and/or anywhere along the spine. Or it might cause headaches. This is very common in patients who have suffered head trauma after falls. Patients can even get headaches many years after wearing orthodontic braces!

But the symptoms of SD aren't limited to pain. SD can cause irritability and/or the inability to think clearly ("brain fog"), as well as organ problems such as digestive, bladder, and even cardiovascular issues. The underlying physiologic cause of SD is unbalanced or increased tissue tension, which in turn impairs either the movement or the function of the different body parts. We call these tight areas "restrictions."

Restrictions can occur in the muscles, joints, fascia, bones, internal organs, and even the seamlike sutures between the bones of the skull and face. They tend to come about after physical trauma or illness or due to asymmetry in the body parts (for instance, leg length differences after joint replacements or after walking with one leg in a cast). They also come about after maintaining abnormal postures for prolonged periods, such as sitting at an improperly configured computer workstation.

Because of complex physical reflexes (viscerosomatic reflexes), organ problems can make the tissues of the nearby trunk and limbs hurt, such as when heart attack pain radiates down the arm or when gallbladder pain refers to the shoulder.

The converse is true too. Body wall problems can affect the function of the adjacent organs (somatovisceral reflexes). Having misaligned pubic bones, for instance, can cause a person to feel "urinary urgency" (as if he has to urinate right away, much like what happens when someone has a bladder infection). It can even cause bed-wetting in children.

The point is, with SD all the body parts—even the organs—are indirectly linked to all the other body parts through soft-tissue connections. Thus, to treat low back pain, an OMM doctor might have to free up restrictions in a distant area such as the ankle or knee, even if those areas don't hurt. It makes sense! If your ankle doesn't bend properly on one side, it's going to indirectly affect how you stand and walk, and in turn your altered posture will affect your back, putting more or less pressure on certain disks and joints.

Recently I treated a man with low back pain using only OMM. He left completely pain-free, and I never touched his low back. I treated only his shoulder, neck, and ribs, as they were the tightest areas on his body—even tighter than his low back, which was the part of him that hurt!

You'll understand the connection if you know anatomy. A muscle called the latissimus dorsi stretches from the low back to the shoulder, and a muscle called the quadratus lumborum connects the bottom of the rib cage to the pelvis, which in turn is connected to the low back through the sacral bone. Thus treating my patient's shoulder and rib cage freed the muscular attachments and loosened up his low back without my directly treating it. Put another way I treated the cause of his problem, not just the symptoms.

Don't Confuse MPS and SD
With Fibromyalgia

Just to be clear, MPS and SD are entirely different from fibromyalgia (FM). Unlike MPS and SD, which I can objectively prove patients have by examining them with my hands and feeling the areas of restricted motion and/or tissue texture changes, FM is a "diagnosis of exclusion." I can't actually prove a person has it because their tissue and movement feel normal to me. I can only prove they don't have other disorders by running lab tests, and then I can guess they might have FM because I didn't find anything else wrong with them.

Real cases of fibromyalgia seem to be associated with other "rheumatologic" conditions such as rheumatoid arthritis and lupus. However, in my opinion fibromyalgia is overdiagnosed, not underdiagnosed. That means people are told they have it when they really have something else—such as MPS, SD, emotional issues, sleep disruption, lack of exercise, or some combination of the above.

The physical examination is also how we distinguish MPS from fibromyalgia. If a person has fibromyalgia, a doctor's pressing on the knots ("tender points") causes pain only over the knots. In contrast, if a person has MPS, pressing on the knots ("trigger points") causes him to feel pain in a much wider and/or distant area. With MPS, pressing on point A causes the patient to hurt at points A and B. With fibromyalgia, pressing on point A causes the individual to hurt only at point A.

How to Find Specialists in SD

Unfortunately it is exceedingly unlikely that an "allopathic" medical doctor (an MD) in *any* specialty, including my own, has the required training to identify SD. That's because in traditional medical schools we MDs don't learn about SD. It's a diagnosis that doctors of osteopathy (DO) are more likely to make, as DOs are required to learn about SD in their medical school training.

The reason I (a medical doctor) know about SD and OMM (the treatment for SD) is that I live in a geographical area that is relatively rich in OMM specialists. Hence, about ten years ago when I had back pain, I went to OMM clinicians for conservative treatment and had a great outcome. From then on I was hooked, both personally and professionally. Since that time I have taken eight hundred hours of course work in OMM both locally and at Harvard University.

However, just because a physician is a DO, that doesn't mean he or she necessarily knows how to recognize or treat SD. Unfortunately most DO students and residents don't retain the required skills they learn in school, as that knowledge gets buried under a heap of other information that comes later. I've heard estimates that as few as only 10 percent to 20 percent of DOs treat SD in their practices.

That's why when my patients move out of state, I suggest they find doctors who are board-certified in OMM. I think it's better to go to a doctor who specializes in utilizing these skills rather than one who only dabbles in it.

To find out more about somatic dysfunction or to locate a manual medicine doctor in your geographical area, visit www.academyofosteopathy .org. If you don't find a link that leads to a doctor in your area, you can always call the American Academy of Osteopathy directly and ask for practitioners' names.

With regard to the techniques the different doctors utilize, let me say a few words about high velocity low amplitude (HVLA) techniques. These techniques can be similar to methods chiropractors use. The doctor will find joints that are not moving as well as they should and use quick thrusts to break through that barrier. It's not uncommon for patients to hear a popping noise. I personally don't like those techniques as much as the gentler, "indirect," unwinding-type techniques, though I admit HVLA is more useful for treating certain conditions, and I occasionally use it too, except for in the head and neck areas.

The main problem I see with HVLA is that patients often feel out of control and vulnerable and have trouble relaxing, knowing they are going to be popped, even if the techniques can be helpful when properly administered. So if you're a tightly wound person who has trouble relaxing, you might prefer a doctor who uses gentler "indirect" techniques.

Do you want even more practical advice? (My gosh, I'm literally spoon-feeding you here.) As you search for an OMM doctor in your area, ask the following questions to the nurses and medical assistants, and do it over the phone *before* you schedule your first appointment. Basically interview the doctors' office staff over the phone and choose your best option depending on their answers.

If the nurses you speak with don't know the answers, have them ask the doctors when it's convenient and get back with you with the answers. You might even make it easy on everybody and fax your questions or drop them off at the office so the nurses don't have to write them down. You want the nurses to like you, right? Make their lives easier and you'll be golden. Here are the questions you should ask.

- Is your doctor board-certified *specifically in OMM*? (Don't just ask if the doctor is "board-certified" without specifying the OMM part.)

- What percentage of the time does your doctor use HVLA (popping and cracking)? (Less of that would be better for anxious or tightly wound patients.)

- Does he or she screen the whole body or just jump right in and treat the area that hurts? (Screening the whole body would be better.)

- Does he or she do craniosacral OMM and treat ribs? (If the answer is no, try a different doctor. These areas commonly contribute to pain and should be addressed.)

- What percentage of the day does your doctor spend doing OMM? (All day is the best answer.)

As you can see, this SD condition is difficult to diagnose because so few clinicians have experience with it. But if you persevere, you can find the treatment you need. You just have to be your own advocate and never give up.

Manual Physical Therapists

If you don't have access to DOs in your area who specialize in OMM, which will likely be the case if you don't live near a school for osteopathic medicine, let me give you another option: call around to your local physical therapy facilities and ask if they have "manual physical therapists" (manual PTs) on staff.

Manual physical therapists are a subset of physical therapists who receive additional training in manual medicine. Generally they don't learn much about it in PT school (it's the same with doctors). They usually learn it in a piecemeal way by going to weekend courses.

Many manual PTs learn osteopathic methods at their courses, so their treatment can be as effective as (or more effective than) the treatment you might receive from a DO, especially if the PT is skilled at what Dr. Stiles calls "sequencing" and finding the "key lesion," or "area of greatest restriction."

If the facilities do have manual therapists on staff, call ahead and find out if they: (1) treat ribs; (2) "sequence" treatments by screening the whole body (not just the painful area) and treating the tightest areas first, and then the next tightest, and so forth, according to Dr. Stiles's sequencing methods; and (3) perform craniosacral OMM.

While physical therapists who *don't* do these things can still be helpful, those who truly can look for restrictions all over your body, including your ribs and your head, and those who treat your restrictions in the right order can be even more helpful.

Be aggressive (but nice) here. Have the administrative assistants write down your questions and read them back to you before they show the paper to the PTs. Or ask to speak with the PTs directly so you can get the answers firsthand. Too much gets lost in translation when you relay complicated language like this over the phone.

If the PTs you call don't know what these questions even mean—if in response to your questions, they say, "What's craniosacral OMM?" or "Huh? What do you mean 'treat ribs'?"—call a different facility, even if that means you have to drive out of your way for treatment. If you have limited resources for travel, at least choose a "manual PT" over a regular PT.

What About Chiropractic Medicine?

By now you might have noticed that I left chiropractic medicine out of this discussion. I did that because I know more about Dr. Stiles's method of OMM and manual PT than I do about chiropractic, and naturally I favor the techniques I know about. That's just human nature.

But beyond that, I have to judge from what the patients tell me. The vast majority who experience both chiropractic medicine and OMM (especially Dr. Stiles's sequenced treatments) tell me they prefer OMM. They say that with Dr. Stiles's type of OMM, fewer treatments are required to get the relief to "stick."

Patients also say the results seem more permanent. With chiropractic (and also with regular physical therapy), patients are generally treated several times a week for many months, and then the pain sometimes returns after treatment ends. Again, Dr. Stiles might say that the recurrence of pain could be due to the clinician not recognizing the main area of hindrance or restriction (for instance, if your low back hurts, chiropractors and PTs tend to treat your low back first, when the "key area" might be your ribs or your shoulders).

However, with that being said, use common sense. There could be patients who feel the opposite way. For all I know, they could be telling their chiropractor that OMM doesn't work because their OMM practitioner didn't sequence their treatments correctly either. Again, it's a matter of perspective, right? None of us sees the whole picture the way God sees it.

That's why you must use common sense. If your chiropractor is helping, keep going as long as your family doctor agrees. Properly executed chiropractic treatment absolutely does seem to help at least a subgroup of people and definitely has its role in the world of manual medicine. Plus, it costs less per visit and is easier to find, even in remote, rural areas. Thus, it may be your only reasonable option anyway.

Finally, check with your family doctor to make sure it's safe for you to undergo treatment by any of us manual medicine clinicians. If your bones are brittle or you're medically fragile, your doctor might say no. Only a doctor who knows you well and who knows the reputation of the manual medicine specialists in your area can safely make that decision for you.

Doctors Can't Give You What They Don't Have

On a final note in this chapter, if you do end up having SD or MPS and find yourself getting upset that your doctor didn't discover it sooner, I challenge you to let it go. The truth is, no matter how many years it took you to find your answer, you're one of the blessed few who ever finds relief. Most people never get diagnosed and treated properly because so few doctors and PTs are taught about these conditions in the first place! For all you know, your doctors might even have the same condition and not know about their options either!

The better way to handle this is: (1) get evaluated and, if appropriate, properly treated by an expert in SD; and (2) after you get better, tell your medical doctors how much the OMM treatment helped. Instead of grumbling about how broken the current medical system is, do something to make it better. Be part of a grassroots effort to educate people (especially your medical doctors) about the potential benefits of OMM.

Maybe after hearing your testimony, your doctors will send other patients for earlier treatment—even if they don't exactly understand what "those OMM doctors" (like me) actually do. Just think of all the people you could keep out of unnecessary surgery!

Word-of-mouth testimonies are the key here. I used to try to "preach" to my medical colleagues about the benefits of OMM, but it didn't work. My patients (who were sent to me by their friends) had to tell their doctors about it to convince them.

As I close this chapter, let me tell you a rather funny story along these lines. For a while, I actually prayed to God that my MD colleagues might get small but treatable cases of SD so I could treat them, get them better, and hence convince them of the benefits of OMM. But when I relayed the story about this prayer to my friend, Dr. Ross Pope (a wonderful OMM specialist in my area who treats me every month), he said, "Rita, that's not a prayer. That's a *curse*." I immediately repented of my poor choice of words and, thankfully, God gave me a *much* better way of getting the word out about SD and MPS. You're reading it right now!

ACTION POINT
Questions to Ask God in Prayer

✧ Lord, do I carry emotional and spiritual tension in my physical body? If so, in what body part or through what symptoms do I express conflict?

✧ At those times when I feel tension, will You give me a healthy method or outlet so I can release my tension to You? Or just take it away without my understanding what it was?

✧ Is my problem due to hidden sin? Unforgiveness? A lie that I believe about myself? Lord, I am sorry for my sin [name it], and I totally and completely forgive [fill in the blank], with no expectation of apology or remediation.

✧ Lord, is there an important physical problem that my other doctors missed? If I do have a physical problem, will You help me find someone who can treat me?

Chapter 6

SOMETIMES YOUR SENSES LIE

MAYBE I'M A little abrupt, but within a few minutes of meeting new patients and visually examining them, I'm already touching them for the physical exam. I prefer to hear the rest of their medical history while I have my hands on them. I learn more through my hands than I do through my eyes and ears some days.

When I met Sandy, I had to modify my approach. I could clearly feel that I made her nervous. I found her skin to be cold and clammy, and the more I touched her neck, the more she tensed up. I figured she was just afraid that I'd hurt her, since she already hurt there. That's understandable.

On that first visit it was clear that I wasn't going to be able to work on her. I could feel her body fighting me, and if I forced things, she'd hurt worse. So to gain her trust, I put her in physical therapy with a good friend of mine. I figured that maybe a few hot pack and electrical stimulation treatments plus my PT friend's excellent OMM skills and bedside manner would help Sandy relax enough to be more treatable.

At that time I didn't know anything about Sandy's past. It took a few months for the therapist and me to figure things out. Sandy's first husband was a volatile man who regularly dragged Sandy around by her hair and/or grabbed her at the neck and bashed her head into walls. Part of her neck pain was due to the physical injuries he caused her, and another part of her neck pain was due to the emotional burden she was carrying in her neck as a result of the abuse.

This is another example of how, whether you are consciously aware of your memories or not, they can manipulate you through a sight, a smell, or even a physical touch to a body part. If somebody touches you in a place that you have infused with strong emotion, like your head and neck in my patient's case, it can stress you out and lead you to stress eat or into some other stress-induced behavior. Or it can trigger physical pain or flare-ups of other physical illness.

Just as lies from the past can cause stress that leads to unhealthy behaviors and choices, sensory stimulation can do the same. In this chapter I discuss how your senses can trigger stress by conjuring up subconscious memories from your past. When you discover how your senses can mislead you, you become more cautious in how you interpret them.

Physical Touch, Memories, and Unwanted Emotion

Physical touch and past memories can be connected, especially if those memories are emotionally charged. On being touched in areas that are meaningful to them, patients remember events that they had forgotten for years—losses, injuries, abandonment, disappointments, etc.

Here's what my patient Andy said: "Gee, Doc, when you started working on my arm, I remembered that time I fell off my bike when I was seven. I had to go to the emergency room and get stitches on my elbow. I was so scared. All I remember is my dad and one of their orderlies holding me down and my mom crying like I was going to die."

Andy remembered the event vividly, even though he was now over fifty years old. In fact, with my hands on his body I could feel him tense up as though he actually relived those emotions from the past.

Patients like Andy sometimes have "somato emotional releases" during treatment. The word *somatic* means "body," so the word "somato emotional" means emotions are being released through the body due to the physical touch from the examiner. Patients literally break down and sob out loud, or they simply release heat from their emotionally charged body parts without awareness of any emotion. Andy did the latter. I could feel his elbow get hot as I worked on him.

No matter how the patients release their pent-up emotional tension, it's not unusual for their tight joints to suddenly pop or click their way loose afterward, allowing me to continue with the more physical aspects of the patients' treatments. That's why I dialogue with pain patients about emotional issues. They loosen up in both ways, mentally and physically, and I am able to do more to help them.

The Limbic System

Some clinicians, including my mentor, Ed Stiles, DO, think this mind-body, emotional-physical connection is mediated by the part of the brain known as the limbic system. In a sense the limbic system acts as an integrator of signals coming from the person's emotions and his or her physical body. Because you have a limbic system, your emotions can trigger physical responses, and physical sensations such as pain can trigger emotions.

Dr. Stiles is probably right, because in the world of pain-management research many studies on pain and emotions agree with his theory. The limbic system part of your brain "lights up" on PET scan research studies that connect physical pain and emotions.

Knowing how the limbic system connects your emotions and your physical tension should actually give you hope. You can literally "will" your body to relax, and you can focus on positive thoughts that lead to positive emotions. You have control over both types of information your limbic system processes. You can literally rewire your brain pathways to fire in a healthier way if you choose the right thoughts and actions.

When you're emotionally tense, you're physically tense too. Just think about how you hike your shoulders up next to your ears when you're stressed. Or think about how you grip the steering wheel until your knuckles turn white when you're driving and are late getting to your destination. On the other hand, when you relax and drop your shoulders, or when you force your fingers to relax your grip on the steering wheel, your whole body relaxes and your mind relaxes too.

Now for the practical teaching point: because physical triggers cause you to reexperience stressful emotions and memories from the past, they can trigger you to reach for false comforters to medicate your unpleasant emotions as well as your physical pain. Thus, if you feel the urge to drink alcohol, overeat, smoke, etc., check your level of physical tension. If you are physically tense and are holding your shoulders up next to your ear lobes, get away from whatever (or whoever) is tempting you. Pray instead. Fill your mind with thoughts that relax you and find a physical position that helps you to release tension. It's never too late to retrain your limbic system.

My Own Molecules of Emotion

During a session in which my arm was being manipulated, I suddenly experienced overwhelming fear and felt as if I were being taken somewhere that I didn't want to go. I had repressed this traumatic memory for at least forty years.

When I was three years old, I fell into the hot asphalt that was being laid onto our new driveway. It burned, and so I was scared and in pain at the same time. I don't recall where my parents were, but I remember my older brothers pulling me into the house and then scrubbing the asphalt off of me with kerosene-soaked cloths as I stood in the bathtub, screaming and crying. As you might imagine, I felt very out of control and vulnerable, even though I knew that my brothers were trying to help me.

Research by a famous, highly published and well-respected scientist in pain research named Candace Pert, PhD, sheds further light on this mind-body connection. Dr. Pert was the first researcher to discover the opiate (morphine) receptor. Her work set the stage for what I do as a pain-management doctor, so I have a lot of respect for her.

More recently Dr. Pert discovered memory receptors and receptors that are involved in the processing of emotions—but she found them outside the brain. She actually found them in *non*-nervous tissue in the body, such as the tissue of the arms and legs. She talks about this in her book *Molecules of Emotion*.[1]

As a result of these amazing findings Dr. Pert postulated that memory and emotions are stored in bodily tissues outside the brain. If she's right, that might explain why some of my patients don't recall previously forgotten past traumatic experiences until I actually touch their emotionally charged body parts during manipulation.

Smells, Memories, and Unwanted Emotions

Are there certain smells that remind you of people or events from your past? In my case it's the smell of the fresh tomato puree and fresh basil. To this day I get the warm fuzzies when I smell tomatoes and basil because it reminds me of my parents and of my distinctly Italian childhood.

It makes sense anatomically and physiologically that smells conjure up memories and emotions. All three are stored in the same part of the brain I just told you about: the limbic system. In fact, the sense of smell is supposed to be the strongest sense associated with memory, even more than sights, sounds, and physical touch.

That's why you have to be careful when you smell something that brings back negative memories. Certain smells can give you the warm fuzzies, but if the smell conjures up fear, anger, depression, or other unwanted emotions, you might be tempted to stress eat to allay those unwanted thoughts and feelings.

For example, if you smell burning wood and it reminds you of the house fire in which you lost a family member, then you might become anxious or angry and feel driven to reach for false comforters to calm your unpleasant emotions. Perhaps the smell will stir up a feeling of loss or remind you of the fear you personally experienced as a result of the fire. The smell might even make your heart pound and race because it reminds you so strongly of the traumatic event.

Or perhaps Christmas smells such as cinnamon and apples or the smell of a pine tree remind you of when your mother died on Christmas Eve. Maybe that causes you to feel tremendous grief that might otherwise lead you to eat as an escape from those emotions.

Or maybe you smell the cologne of a person who abused you in the past (perhaps it's Eau de' Beer), and you have a flashback to those times when you felt vulnerable under the control of that person. That smell could indirectly trigger you to reach for your false comforter.

Because smells trigger memories and emotions, it's important for you to take inventory of how you feel when exposed to those smells that you identify as your triggers. Then remind yourself that your emotions do not rule you. Sometimes just identifying the source of the unwanted emotions helps you find relief.

Sights and Emotions

Sandy, my patient with the neck issues, nearly fell apart during one of her follow-up appointments. While she was in the waiting room with the other patients, she went to the front desk and asked if there was any way she could be moved into an exam room right away. She said she was on the verge of a panic attack.

When I saw Sandy a while later, my medical assistant had already given me a heads-up about her waiting room scene. I figured it was a divine opportunity to understand why she was so tense and hard to manipulate. So I probed into why she reacted that way.

"Well, I was doing a lot better until a few minutes ago. All of a sudden, when I was in your waiting room, I started getting a headache and my neck pain went crazy."

After a few minutes of dialoguing to find her specific stressor, she realized that she had seen a man who reminded her of her abusive ex-husband, sitting next to a woman with a cast on her broken right arm. At one time her abusive ex broke her right arm, and that sight was a little too close to home for Sandy.

Sandy didn't realize it, but her choice of words revealed even more about her hidden thoughts and emotions. She said her neck pain "went crazy" while she was in the waiting room. After further dialoguing, something clicked and she realized, "I guess I thought I was going to go crazy with fear."

Almost as soon as she realized the source of her added tension, she let out a sigh and was able to let her shoulders fall back down to where they were supposed to be. Her previous fear had caused her shoulders to be pinned up next to her ears. Within a few minutes I was able to get a little done with OMM, and she felt better. But really I think the emotional debriefing helped her more than anything.

This is an example of how the emotional side of you can believe the thought that you are in danger, even though the adult, logical side of you knows that you're not actually in danger.

Your Senses May Lie

A few months ago I had an unexplained low self-esteem day. I felt very unsure of myself, even at work when counseling patients. For some unexplainable reason I felt like I wasn't doing as good of a job as usual, even though I knew logically it was a lie.

This happens to me every now and then, particularly when I'm tired. If I don't get enough sleep, I just feel "blah," and I border on feeling depressed. However, at this particular time, I was well rested. Truly I had no good reason to feel bad about myself. Later that night I figured out what was going on.

During our Wednesday night Eden Diet online chat at www .EdensFreedomSisters.NING.com, I confessed to the ladies that I was feeling low for no obvious reason, and you should have seen what happened. They all swarmed around me like mother hens, trying to boost my self-esteem and help me out of my transient funk. It was really sweet but kind of funny too. I didn't really mind feeling bad, but they were all trying to hard to fix me so I wouldn't have to endure the negative feelings!

That's when it occurred to me that God was using me to minister to them about how negative feelings don't actually kill you. They were going out of their way to help me stop feeling bad (which was sweet of them), but I really didn't ask for or need the rescue. As I chatted with them, God gave me the clear message to pass on to them, "Just because you feel bad, it doesn't mean you *are* bad. Sometimes your feelings lie to you."

Apparently a couple of these women had an extreme aversion to dealing with negative emotions, which is probably why they turned to food so often for consolation. These ladies needed to see that it was OK to feel those negative emotions. When I told them that, one of the women said, "This too shall pass." It was like she had an epiphany.

They also needed to see that I could have low self-esteem days after I lost weight. They needed to see that you're not always on cloud nine after you lose weight, even if you're a doctor. Weight loss (and being a doctor) does not equal "constant euphoria."

The next time you have a low self-esteem day, remember, "This too shall pass." You don't need to reach for a false comforter to escape those emotions. Your senses sometimes lie to you. Just because you feel bad doesn't mean you *are* bad.

As I said before, emotions and logic do not necessarily communicate with each other. That's why it's important to dissect your thoughts and emotions down to their roots. Once you do that, you can more easily identify the wrong thoughts that led to your negative emotions and reject them.

ACTION POINT
Questions to Ask God in Prayer

✧ Lord, will You help me realize if certain sensory experiences trigger my unwanted emotions?

✧ Lord, if I can't hear Your answer, is it because I am up against a barrier that I created, which prevents me from hearing You?

✧ What is the nature of my barrier? Do I believe a lie about myself, You, others, or a situation or event? Or is something else blocking me from hearing You or remembering what You want me to remember?

✧ Do I need to deal with sin in my life to get through this barrier, or forgive somebody? Lord, I totally and completely forgive [fill in the blank] with no expectation of apology or remediation. Or is something else blocking me from hearing You right now? If I'm not getting an answer, will You please come through, over, or under my barrier to help me anyway?

PART THREE

THE SPIRITUAL YOU
Seeing Through God's Eyes

Chapter 7

THE ACCUSER

U P TO THIS point we've been talking about the interrelationship between mind, body, and spirit. If any one of those areas of your life lacks your attention and care, *the whole you* suffers. Though we've reviewed a multitude of problems that can plague your mind and body, the primary obstacle standing in the way of your health and happiness is a spiritual one. Specifically it's a guy I call the accuser. You may know him as the devil.

To get a better understanding of just who the accuser is and what he tries to do, let's look at a few passages of Scripture:

> [The devil] was a murderer from the beginning, not holding to the truth, for there is no truth in him. When he lies, he speaks his native language, for he is a liar and the father of lies.
>
> —JOHN 8:44

> Put on the full armor of God so that you can take your stand against the devil's schemes. For our struggle is not against flesh and blood, but against the rulers, against the authorities, against the powers of this dark world and against the spiritual forces of evil in the heavenly realms.
>
> —EPHESIANS 6:11-12

> Your enemy the devil prowls around like a roaring lion looking for someone to devour.
>
> —1 PETER 5:8

I think you get the picture. Murderer, liar, schemer, evil—these are the words that best describe our spiritual enemy, who is dedicated to bringing us down. This is why I like to call our erroneous internalized beliefs "lies." I believe the accuser has a hand in them. He wants us to believe misinformation, particularly if it's destructive.

The accuser combines these lies with a myriad of other weapons at his disposal: greed, pride, lust, shame, guilt, envy, bitterness, laziness, anger, and fear to name a few. He's an expert at deploying them all against us.

Take another look at that last verse above. The devil is like a lion. Have you ever watched lions on a hunt? They don't even try to face off against the biggest and fastest gazelles on the Serengeti. No, they hide in the tall grass and watch for the smallest, slowest, and weakest members of the herd. These are the ones the lions attack.

What I'm saying is that kids are prime targets for the accuser. They are innocent, and they lack experience and perspective with which to police and correct their perceptions. They make easy prey. And not that he stops with children—he does plenty of damage to us grownups too.

Whether taking on kids or adults, the accuser is a master at distorting our beliefs—often for years and sometimes for a lifetime. Fortunately we have a Savior who can knock that charlatan back where he belongs and reveal the true picture of who we are. Let's take a closer look at what the accuser is up to, what that means for our physical and emotional health, and what we can do about it.

Feeling Like a Hypocrite

Cindy is a thirty-year-old youth minister's wife and lives in Small Town, USA. She wears a kind of mask to convince people that she is happy and fulfilled in her church position. She even fools herself into believing it some of the time. But when I sorted through her physical and emotional problems to find the source of her headaches, I learned the truth about her.

Cindy feels like a complete hypocrite as a youth pastor's wife. She believes she doesn't deserve to be a role model for teenagers because of all the bad, ungodly things she did when she was a youth. She got pregnant at age seventeen and had an abortion without telling her parents. She got pregnant again at age nineteen but had the baby and gave it up for adoption. Her parents found out and made her do it.

Sadly Cindy wasn't able to conceive again after that, even when she was happily married to the youth minister. Due to the repeated and untreated STDs from her teenage years, her fallopian tubes scarred shut.

Not surprisingly Cindy suffered with a triple dose of guilt later on in life. She felt unforgivable due to the abortion, she felt like a bad and uncaring mother for giving up her second baby, and she felt like a bad wife for not being able to have a baby for her loving preacher-husband.

Any way she looked at herself, she judged herself as bad, dirty, shameful, and a worthless hypocrite. She believed this despite the fact that she knew Scripture and realized (intellectually) that God forgave her. Just like innumerable other patients I've counseled, what she knew intellectually and what she felt emotionally didn't line up.

In a sense I can relate to Cindy's past. I was overweight and didn't date until I was much older than average (after I lost the weight), but I still judged myself as bad or good, and I still felt guilt over certain things. As a result I used to think like this, "Was I good today? No, I was bad. I ate a piece of candy. Am I a good person? No, I gained a pound; therefore I am bad, fat, and disgusting." Or, "Yay! I lost five pounds! I'm going to celebrate by eating fried cheese sticks!"

Even now if I overeat at times (trust me, it still happens), I'm tempted to feel like a hypocritical diet doctor. "I should be totally over this by now!" Wrong. I'm still human. I still have very stressful days. My life is not a piece of cake (sorry, I couldn't resist the pun or the cake) all of the time. The accuser is continually whispering lies to us that cause us to judge ourselves and others and that lead us to stress eat or to fall into equally harmful behaviors. He also works hard at disrupting our most important relationships.

I SEE You

When I first watched the movie *Avatar*, I was struck by the way the large, blue alien Na'vi people greeted one another. They said, "I see you."[1] However, they didn't mean, "I see what you look like." They meant, "I see the essence of the real you, deep-down, beyond your exterior. You're worth looking at."

Don't we all have the need to be seen and accepted on a deep level for who we are? I believe God implanted us with the desire for real relationship exactly so we would turn to Him to fill that need. When our need for fellowship and connection isn't met, we turn to counterfeit sources of fulfillment, such as false comforters.

When one of my patients, a woman named Angela, was young, she didn't experience anything close to deep, relational, "I see you" understanding and acceptance from her parents. She recalled that her mother walked around in an emotional fog, and her father believed in the "little children should be seen but not heard" philosophy.

Because of the frustration and anxiety Angela felt about not being heard or truly *seen* by her parents, she ate. No matter how disconnected she felt from her parents or from her emotions, she always felt connected to food. Food always understood her.

Angela recalled her mother saying, "Why are you so overly sensitive?" rather than, "I understand," on those rare times that Angela approached her, upset. At times her mother (because of her own baggage) would talk right over Angela, as if to say, "I don't even hear you talking to me. I'm putting no effort into hearing you. I'm looking at you, but I don't see you."

Angela said her mom was not a communicator, and she was strongly ruled by shame and fear, so she didn't talk much about her anxiety. However, Angela could see it in her shaking hands and her "deer-in-headlights" panicky demeanor, which got much, much worse as she grew older. I think the accuser was working overtime in that household—not only on Angela but also on her parents.

Whether it's due to your parent's anxiety, mental illness, past traumatic events, or mind-altering medicines, having a parent who isn't able to "connect" with you can do a number on your self-esteem. It can even cause you to feel anxious. As a result you can learn to run from your emotions or bury them in food, just as Angela did. Obviously this doesn't happen to everybody with anxiety, but I've seen it happen in some.

The "I'm Bad" Lie

Because the flesh makes us egocentric (instead of God-centered), our default mode is to draw conclusions based on our self-centeredness. If something bad happens—even if it has nothing to do with us—we think like Steve Urkel from the old TV sitcom *Family Matters*, "Did I do that?"[2]

Then we conclude almost automatically on the subconscious level, "I'm the one who caused this problem. It's entirely my fault. I'm just bad."

There are too many "I'm bad" lies to name, but for your sake let me name a few common ones. "I am bad because I drink," "I'm bad because I'm fat," "I'm bad because I look at porn," "I am bad; therefore, I was abandoned," and "I'm bad because I was sexually abused."

Don't forget these: "Because I am bad, nobody loves me. God doesn't even love me and won't hear or answer my prayers. He is too disgusted with me." Or, "I must have done something really bad to be punished with this problem." Or, "Because of my disfigurement, I'm ruined for life. The only way I can keep others away from hurting me is to insulate myself with [a layer of fat or mind-altering drugs]."

These subconscious lies make us nervous. We feel threatened by them. Thus we turn to our false comforters for relief. "Something bad is going to happen because I am bad. I'm afraid. I might as well have some more chocolate, since that usually takes my mind off my bad self for a while. But, hey, thank God I'm not as bad as those drug addicts. At least my addiction is legal. (Enter pride)."

It's possible to respond differently to the "I'm bad" anxiety. Your outward actions might even seem "good" in response to the lie. But your motives are wrong. You think, "Because I am bad, I must constantly do good works so I can try to become good. What should I take on as my next project?"

Instead of reaching for false comforters, reach for the real Comforter, the Holy Spirit. In Hebrews 10 the Holy Spirit spoke about the things that make us feel that we're bad. He said, "Their sins and lawless acts I will remember no more" (v. 17).

The author of Hebrews went on to say, "And where these have been forgiven, there is no longer any sacrifice for sin" (v. 18). In other words, you don't have to keep doing good works to make up for whatever you think makes you a bad person.

The "I'm a Bad Doctor" Lie

If you think doctors are immune to believing lies about themselves, think again. Not too long ago I gave one of my favorite patients a shot in his low back, and five days later he lost sensation in his legs.

At first I did the Steve Urkel thing, "Oh no! What did I do wrong?" I replayed the procedure at least fifty times in my mind and couldn't find my mistake. As I waited for the MRI results, I was convinced I would find an infection. It was the only thing that made sense, given the five-day gap.

After spending a gazillion insurance dollars on additional blood work, a spinal tap, and three other MRIs (not to mention spending my own energy on worrying and experiencing false guilt), it turned out my patient had multiple sclerosis (MS) much higher up in his spine, where I didn't even touch him. The timing of the MS exacerbation and the shot in his low back was entirely coincidental.

There is no way anyone but God Himself could have known that my patient had MS until it became worse and declared itself. Still, just like Steve Urkel, I believed it had something to do with what *I* did—me, me, me! As if I'm somehow the center of the universe.

Thankfully God used this situation to teach me. He said, "You can't let one false alarm in eight years of giving spinal injections scare you like that. You have to continue to try to help people, even if I don't tell you everything that's wrong with all patients when you first meet them."

My friend, you can't let fear, worry, and self-condemnation stand in your way either—not even for a minute. You have to keep trying to help people, no matter what the accuser tells you.

Self-Punishment

I was in college and having a very bad day. I don't remember exactly what negative thought or emotion triggered my self-hatred. Maybe I felt out of control over my weight. Or maybe I got a lower grade than I expected on a test. It could even have been a case of unrequited love. You know how those college dating soap operas go.

The only thing I remember for sure is the "aha" moment during an eating binge when I realized, "Oh my gosh, I'm stuffing myself to the point of feeling sick in order to punish myself!"

Being young and not having gone to medical school yet, I didn't know anyone who cut themselves or burned themselves with cigarettes. I didn't even know "self-punishment" behavior existed. Yet instinctively I began to wonder if I was trying to punish myself by overeating.

Why would I want to punish myself by bingeing? I didn't consciously think I deserved punishment. If anything I was doing all the right things. I lost a substantial amount of weight, I was attending an Ivy League university, I was (overall) a "good" girl with the boys, and I did my homework. Other students went out several nights a week partying, and I was the boring one who actually did what I was supposed to do. Why did I deserve punishment?

With the benefit of hindsight and maturity I can now look back at that event and understand perfectly what was going on in my subconscious mind. Clearly whatever had been going on in my life at the time stirred up my deep-seeded, childhood "I'm bad" complex. No matter how many good things I accomplished, they weren't enough to erase my deep-down belief that I was in some way defective and deserving of punishment. You can't erase one lie (that you're lowly) with another lie (that you can make yourself worthy through good works).

Please let me take a moment to vindicate my family. Don't assume that it was their fault that I had low self-esteem as a child. My parents had their quirks (as we all do), but they definitely were not verbally abusive toward me. In fact, I distinctly remember my mother saying (in Italian), "Whatever she applies herself to, she does well."

Does that sound like a message that would cause a child to have low self-esteem? Mostly my self-esteem issues sprang out of my own, judgmental head, probably from direct accusations by the evil little snake.

Self-Judgment

The next time you're tempted to weigh yourself to determine if you're "good" or "bad" (i.e., to judge yourself as Satan wants you to do), think about the story of when David was tempted by Satan to number the men in his army.

> Satan rose up against Israel and incited David to take a census of Israel. So David said to Joab and the commanders of the troops, "Go and count the Israelites from Beersheba to Dan. Then report back to me so that I may know how many there are." But Joab replied, "May the LORD multiply his troops a hundred times over. My lord the king, are they not all my lord's subjects? Why does my lord want to do this? Why should he bring guilt on Israel?"
>
> —1 CHRONICLES 21:1-3

First, notice that Satan tempted David to count his men. It wasn't God's idea. Therefore you have to conclude that it was some kind of trap. Second, Joab said David ought to feel guilt over it, which further suggests that it was an actual sin.

As far as what kind of sin, I believe it was pride and vanity—maybe even idolatry. It was like David was looking into a mirror while flexing his big, bulging muscles, saying, "How big is my army? *Grrrr!* It's very big!" (Just like his ego.)

He put his pride and his faith in himself rather than God.

You Have to Know What You Are to Know What You're Not

Maybe you're like David in a way. But instead of counting your humongous army, you count your money and possessions. Or maybe you weigh yourself on the bathroom scale to measure your worth. "Am I 'good' or am I 'bad' today? Let me weigh myself to find out."

When you're tempted to weigh yourself for the wrong motives (to measure and judge your worth when you feel unsure of yourself), say out loud, "No! I am *not* what I weigh. I no longer trust human judgments of whether I'm good or bad, and I no longer base my worth on the numbers on the scale!"

That brings me to the next point. If you are not what you weigh, then what are you? You have to know who and what you are to know who and what you're not! When the accuser lies to you and says, "You're bad, you're worthless, you're weak, you're stupid," how are you supposed to know he's lying unless you know what you truly are to begin with? You have to have some standard to compare the lies to, or you won't recognize them as lies. That's what I talk about in the next chapter. I tell you the truth about who you are.

ACTION POINT

Questions to Ask God in Prayer

✷ Lord, are there lies that I might have told myself or lies that others told me about my identity?

✷ Was there judgment mixed into the lies? If so, I'm sorry for my part in it.

✷ What or who do You say I am, Lord? How do You feel about me?

✷ If I can't hear You, is it because I believe a lie about myself, You, others, or a situation? If so, what is the lie? And what is the truth to replace it? Or is there something else blocking me? Will You please come to me and help me despite my barrier?

Chapter 8

YOU ARE DELIGHTFUL

I**N HIS BOOK** *The Man in the Mirror* Patrick Morley wrote about a father and son who flew by seaplane with two other men to a secluded Alaskan bay for a day of fishing. When the group set to take off the next morning, the plane would fly only in a low, circular pattern. They soon realized one of the pontoons had been punctured and was filling with water.

Before long the plane crashed into the water and capsized. All the passengers were alive, but they couldn't locate any safety equipment. So they prayed and then jumped into the icy bay to swim to shore. The four swam against the strong riptide. Two of the men finally reached the shore, exhausted. When they looked back, they saw Phil and his twelve-year-old son, Mark, on the horizon, arm-in-arm, being swept out to sea. The men knew Phil could have made it to shore, and they figured Mark just wasn't a strong enough swimmer. But Phil wasn't going to leave his boy behind. He chose to die with his son than live without him.[1]

The Lord's love for *you* is the same. Regardless of what the accuser tells you, and no matter what you did in the past, God delights in you exactly as you are at this moment—imperfections, mistakes, and all. And He delights in you so much that He would die for you: "For God so loved the world that he gave his one and only Son, that whoever believes in him shall not perish but have eternal life" (John 3:16).

If you want to live more joyfully and freely, then let me help you believe what God says about you in Scripture as you proceed through this chapter and the rest of the book.

Connecting Head and Heart

Some of us who believe and trust in the Lord may quote Psalm 139:14, saying we are fearfully and wonderfully made, or Deuteronomy 28:13, saying we are the head and not the tail. But at the same time on an emotional level we go on feeling bad.

Although our body parts are interconnected and interdependent, we act as though our brains are disconnected from our hearts. Even when we logically know the truth as God says it, we continue to believe the deep down "I'm [bad, worthless, stupid, etc.]" lies.

This was Lonny's experience too. He used to quote Scripture to me, but I had a gut feeling he didn't thoroughly believe what he was saying. Near the end of his high school years Lonny experienced major trauma when his little brother died unexpectedly from an allergic reaction to a bee sting. In response Lonny turned to over-eating to manage his emotions. Within four years he ballooned to over four hundred pounds.

As we dialogued about his early relationship with his family, Lonny mentioned that he was the middle child. His siblings had talents and special attributes that set them apart, but Lonny had no special identity as a child. He felt invisible compared to his little brother and older sister. In a way he even resented his siblings for it.

When his brother died, Lonny just started eating. My guess is he did that in part to become more "visible" and "grounded," when deep down he felt unimportant and unworthy of attention. I wouldn't be surprised if he even felt guilty about having resented his little brother before he died because he seemed more special (being the baby of the family). However, I never got a chance to find out what lies Lonny believed. I had to send him to a surgeon to have a hip replacement, and I never saw him again.

I think Lonny knew intellectually that he was just as special and important as his brother and sister. His heart just didn't believe it.

How Your Memories With
Negative Emotion Are Stored

Let me try to explain this head-heart disconnect in the way a good friend of mine once described it. In some ways your mind is like a computer. It has different file folders representing memories from different times in your life.

If you suffered childhood verbal, physical, or sexual abuse, there's a folder for that. If you were abandoned or neglected, there's a folder for that. If you suffered a loss of a family member or friend, there's a folder for that too.

There's also an open file that you work out of in your everyday adult life. When you go to church or read the Bible or hear the Word, you store new information in that open file. However, that logical, intellectual information doesn't reach the old files because the old files have been sealed off for protection.

Those folders are entirely separate and don't share information. It's the same way with your Microsoft Word files. To change a Word file, you have to specifically open the file in question and specifically save your new information. Entering information into the current open file does nothing to modify your closed Word files.

Why might you subconsciously wall off your sensitive psychological files? It has to do with shame that you internalized as a result of childhood events. Shame makes you hide from God (i.e., hide from truth), just as shame over eating the forbidden fruit made Adam and Eve hide from God in the garden. The more emotionally threatening you perceive the trauma to be, the more deeply you bury the memory in your system. You protect your weakest link.

As I said previously, children see and interpret traumatic events through the limited reasoning skills that match their ages. They don't see their traumatic events through the wisdom of maturity. Thus their shameful conclusions are often corrupted with lies, just as computer programs can be corrupted with viruses. That's why during childhood we wall off the lies that get triggered later in life.

Here's a tangible example. As a logical, wise adult, you know that if a ten-year-old girl is raped by her uncle, it's her uncle's fault and not the girl's. However, if *you* are the girl we are talking about, even if you know logically that ten-year-old girls don't cause their own rapes, part of you (the ashamed girl trapped in a hidden computer file in your mind) might still feel responsible and hence dirty. That's a lie, but the lie feels so powerful and real to the little girl that it causes her to hide from the One who wants to show her truth.

Like a computer, the mind needs virus-protection software to guard it from harmful lies that can cause it to crash. Think of the truth of God as being like virus-protection software. He purges dangerous contaminants (lies) from your system. But He can't work unless your system *allows* His software to penetrate the hidden, corrupt files.

So pray that God helps you open up your innermost places to the light of His truth. Pray that God helps you to remember the relevant, past traumatic events that are keys to your healing. Ask God to help you differentiate the truth from the lies in your memories that lead you into unhealthy compensatory behaviors. And then open up and let Him in.

I Didn't Feel Worthy

A long time ago when I was in the middle of my compulsive eating disorder, I didn't feel that I was allowed to eat "normal" food that *thin* people ate, such as dessert or junk food. If I ate a little bite of cake, I interpreted it as a failure. Thus I was either "on" a diet, eating perfectly healthily, or "off" the diet, overeating junk. It was feast or famine.

Can *you* relate? Maybe you don't feel you deserve gifts that God wants to give you. Perhaps the accuser speaks to you as he spoke to me back then: "Look at you! You're fat! If you knew how to take care of yourself properly, you wouldn't be in this mess. Just look at that other woman over there. She's thin and beautiful, and so, unlike you, she actually deserves to eat that piece of cake."

If the accuser tells you things such as this, he probably tells you that you don't deserve other good things, either. Your beliefs show in the way you receive compliments. Think about it. How do you react when people compliment you? Do you belittle yourself and shake off the compliment, or do you just say, "Thank you"? Your response says a lot about what you think you deserve.

To break free from the lie that you don't deserve good things, prayerfully locate the lie in the depths of your mind, grab hold of it (take every thought captive), and then compare it to the truth you find in Scripture. God gave Solomon great things, and you can have great things too, such as peace, joy, deep emotional healing, and freedom from pain, illness, and addictions.

The Lie That Women Are Worthless or Inferior

Christian authors John and Stasi Eldredge were on Joyce Meyer's TV show *Enjoying Everyday Life* in 2010, talking about "The Heart of a Woman."[2] On that broadcast John and Stasi addressed the misperception that women are less important or less valuable than men. John said it's not like Eve was inferior to Adam just because she was created second. He said God made women second because they are more complex and beautiful. He pointed out that scientists often talk about how simpler creatures (amoebas and such) were created first, and the most complex and beautiful creatures came along last. Women, then, represent the peak of God's creativity. (I took liberties to paraphrase here.)

Make sure you understand what John said. He didn't imply that the woman is better because she is more complex and beautiful and was made after Adam. He simply made an observation without passing judgment on which gender was better than the other.

Can you imagine if God sat up there in heaven, looking down on Adam and Eve, and said that one gender was superior to the other? As I understand it, He made men and women different because we complement each other. I believe the key to our combating these divisive "who is more important than whom" gender issues is to stop judging and start loving each other as Christ loved the church.

A stay-at-home, homeschooling mom is not better than a brain surgeon because she spends more time with her kids. And the male CEO of the Fortune 500 company is not better than the mom because he drives a more expensive car. Don't fall into the accuser's trap and judge yourself and others with gender-based lies. The judgment is what gets you into trouble. Your worth is not determined by your gender. Your worth is determined by the fact that God sent His only Son to die so that you could be reconciled with Him.

A Tale of Two Visions

As a young woman when things didn't go well in my life or if my self-esteem was running low, I blamed it on my weight. If I didn't have a boyfriend, it was because of my weight. If I had a bad hair day, it was because of my weight. If I got three red traffic lights in a row, it was because I was an *overweight* driver. You get the idea.

As the years passed, I began to wonder if I blamed my weight for more than its fair share. Perhaps my weight problem was just a symptom of something deeper and darker—something more painful than the actual eating disorder, perhaps a memory, emotion, or belief that I felt compelled to medicate with food.

I already knew that feeling vulnerable and out of control had something to do with eating disorders. But why did *I* feel out of control? Did something bad happen in my childhood that I don't remember? Did I internalize a lie about myself? I wanted to know.

I prayed to God for answers but didn't expect my answers to come immediately. Nor did I expect them to come in the form of *two visions*.

Before I go on, let me stop and explain what I mean by the word "vision." I don't mean the John Smith kind of vision that led to the founding of Mormonism and the Church of Jesus Christ of Latter-Day Saints. In case there's any doubt, I disagree with all that. I believe the Bible needs no new information added to it, least of all if I write it.

I'm saying only that through my two visions God helped me understand a principle that is *already* in the Bible. Apparently this principle didn't get through my thick skull the previous five hundred times I read or heard about it.

Now, let me give you another heads-up. In the rest of this chapter I tell you about only the first of the two visions. In a way I leave you hanging. I expose the lie that I once believed without telling you the truth that ultimately replaced it. Don't worry. In the next chapter I tell you the wondrous, freeing second half of the story.

And don't worry if the message doesn't resonate with you. Just because the two visions together were earth-shattering, life-changing revelations for me doesn't mean they will speak to you with the same impact. I like what Oswald Chambers said: "Never make a principle out of your experience: let God be as original with other people as He was with you."[3]

With those disclaimers out of the way, let me get down to business and tell you what happened. One day as I rested alone in our guest room immediately after praying, the peace of God came over me, and I fell into an intensely relaxed state in which I had a daydream of sorts.

During this experience I felt as though my consciousness was split into two parts. I was present as my fully aware adult self, Adult Rita (the person who had just finished praying for answers). But I was also present in another form—a much younger version of myself, who for simplicity I call Embryo Rita.

Maybe you can guess why I call the second person Embryo Rita. In this vision I felt like I went back to the womb and physically became an embryo again. How did I know I was an embryo? I felt an intense urge to curl up into a tiny, tiny ball and cover up with the blanket I had been sitting on, so that even my head was covered. Plus I felt very small, I felt like I was floating, and I saw only darkness.

Even though the split consciousness experience was completely new to me and, frankly, weird, I went along with it anyway. I asked God for answers just before this vision occurred, so I believed this was God's unorthodox way of answering my prayer. Plus I felt complete emotional peace. So I didn't worry—not even when I began to sense Satan's presence off to one side.

As the vision unfolded, Satan spoke two very powerful and damaging words to me. He said, "You're bad." In response I took the bait and turned my head toward him, replying, "I am?" Even my voice felt tiny.

The adult part of me couldn't help but notice the tone in my embryo voice. When I said, "I am?" I sounded totally confused. Embryo Rita had never heard the word *bad* before and truly didn't understand what it meant.

It was a short vision, consisting of only four words: "You're bad" and "I am?"

By then Adult Rita, who was observing quietly in the background of my mind, understood the point of the message: my childhood low self-esteem was not due to my having been obese. It was ultimately a result of my tutoring session with Satan. He first taught me the language of accusation, judgment, and condemnation. I didn't even know what the word *bad* meant until he came around.

Do you see how this answered the question I posed to God? Very early on I internalized the belief in my subconscious mind that I was "bad." Believing this led me to feel anxious and threatened, and, in turn, feeling anxious and threatened led me to eat to medicate my emotions. *Voilà!* My low self-esteem *preceded* my weight problems.

With this information, believe it or not, I felt vindicated. Embryos can't actually do anything wrong. According to Scripture I was conceived in sin (Ps. 51:5) and carried the sins of my predecessors as a burden (Deut. 5:9). However, those things were not actually *my* fault! I didn't know the Lord yet as an embryo!

Can you imagine if God rejected all of us as embryos just because we're conceived in sin? Thankfully He gives us second chances through Jesus Christ. Actually He loves us so much that He gives us at least seventy-times-seven chances. Immediately it was like a huge weight was lifted off my shoulders. The relief was permanent too. The truth really does set you free (when you receive it at a very deep level).

Should This Vision Be Taken Literally?

To be safe, I think God meant my vision to be a figurative illustration to help me understand Scripture, not necessarily something to be taken literally. As you know, God communicates with us in the Bible by telling stories because we can relate better to stories than to abstract truths.

However, some people have said that my vision could be taken literally; i.e., "Satan really could speak to us in the womb." To support their viewpoint, they cite Psalm 139:7, "Where can I go from your [God's] Spirit? Where can I flee from your presence?" Verse 13 says, "For you created my inmost being; you knit me together in my mother's womb." They figure if God can enter the womb and knit us together, maybe the devil can enter the womb and accuse us as well.

It would be interesting to hear what the theologians have to say about this issue. After all, it's important to test the concept against the truth in Scripture. As it says in 1 Thessalonians 5:19-22, "Do not quench the Spirit. Do not despise prophecies. Test all things; hold fast what is good. Abstain from every form of evil" (NKJV). Until we hear from the Bible experts, I think it would be safest to accept only the heart of the message (that Satan is the source of condemnation, judgment, and accusation) and put the rest on the back burner. For sure *that* part of the message is scriptural.

Nonetheless it's tempting to pontificate about other parts of this story. For example, can developing babies think, feel, learn, and remember more than we give them credit for? Apparently while I was in the womb, when my brain was small and undeveloped, I had some ability to communicate. In case you missed that, I said I had very little brain as an embryo, but that didn't stop me from talking to the devil. Some people would argue that I haven't changed a bit (especially after they read my admittedly eccentric embryo story).

Seriously I am forced to consider the scientific evidence as well as ponder the spiritual questions. Even at early stages, developing babies have rudimentary brain structures that process emotions and memory. Those are parts of the "primitive" nervous system, and, as I said, they develop early in gestation. Putting the scientific and spiritual elements together, I am inclined to conclude that developing babies must have some degree of emotional and spiritual consciousness. Stated another way, embryos and fetuses aren't the clueless, emotionless blobs that some people think they are.

Just think about what Elizabeth told her cousin, Mary, when she showed up at her house, pregnant with Jesus: "As soon as the sound of your greeting reached my ears, the baby in my womb leaped for joy" (Luke 1:44). According to the Bible, developing babies feel and process emotions. Therefore it's fair to ask, "Can they process prenatal communication at some level too?"

ACTION POINT
Questions to Ask God in Prayer

✧ Lord, did the accuser lie to me about my identity in my past?

✧ What lies did he tell me about myself, You, others, and situations and events in my life?

✧ Lord, what is the truth that refutes each of those lies?

✧ If I don't hear Your answers, Lord, is it because of some kind of barrier that I put up? If so, what caused the barrier? And will You come to me despite the barrier? Or help me come to Your side of it? Or give me a way to tear it down? Or release it?

Chapter 9

NO MORE JUDGMENT

I F YOU HAVE a tendency to judge yourself or others, or if you're a works-oriented rather than grace-oriented person, you really need to hear this message. It's the second half of the story I started in the last chapter, and it consists of another vision.

Once again I was praying, curled up on my comfy chair, feeling deeply relaxed and seeking answers from God. But this time I wasn't sure of what question to ask. So I looked up to heaven and said, "Tell me more, God! You decide what I need to hear." Wasn't it nice of me to give the Master of the universe free rein like that?

It wasn't long before God took me back to the womb for a second visit. The major difference was this time I didn't actually become my fetus self. I remained in the body of "Adult Me," and I was there simply as a voyeur.

In my vision I could see Fetus Rita floating in a transparent, brightly lit womb right in front of me. I could also see that her back was turned toward me. It felt as though she was hiding. I also felt completely emotionally disconnected from her, like there was some kind of barrier between us—like we weren't even part of the same person.

Fetus Rita knew that I was watching her, but something—maybe shame—kept her from turning around and facing me. Perhaps she still believed the lie the devil told her when she was an embryo—that she was "bad."

In this vision I was profoundly aware of God's presence on my left side. Though I didn't actually see Him, I heard His voice audibly for the first time in my life. He said, "Look at her!" as He directed my attention toward Fetus Rita.

It was extremely helpful for me to hear God speak audibly so I could hear His tone of voice. It was profoundly tender and adoring and revealed that He *delighted* in me. But still I was confused. I *was* looking at Fetus Rita, so why did God keep telling me, "Look at her!" when I was already looking at her? I remember thinking, "I don't understand what I'm supposed to see. She's just a fetus. It's not like she can actually *do* anything."

In my thoughts I "felt" God reprimand me, "No! That's not it! Look at her!"

I looked more intently at Fetus Rita and began to wonder, "Maybe God loves her because she's going to become a doctor, help people's backs, and write Christian books." I could tell God did *not* like what I was thinking. After a brief pause I once again heard God say, "Look at her!" Except now He emphasized the word *look*.

"*Look* at her!"

That's when I finally understood. When God said, "Look at her," He meant something much more profound than I initially realized. He didn't mean look at her with my eyes. He meant "*Look* at her with your heart and *see* what I see. I don't love her because she's going to serve Me. I love her because she's my creation!"

Ignore the Lies. Focus on Truth

Psychologists say that when you reinforce positive behavior and ignore the negative, the negative behaviors automatically "extinguish." They burn themselves out when you don't give them fuel. That's what God did in my vision. He ignored the devil and robbed him of fuel.

In my embryo vision Satan told me I was "bad." But in the fetus vision that followed, God didn't erase the lie by telling me the opposite—that I was "good." In fact, He didn't judge me at all. He just *delighted* in me.

I admit I was disappointed. I wanted to hear God say, "Rita, you're not *bad*. You're *good*!" But it wouldn't have been right for Him to tell me that! If Jesus Himself didn't like being called "good," I surely couldn't be "good" in God's eyes. "'Why do you call me good?' Jesus answered. 'No one is good—except God alone'" (Mark 10:18).

In the same way God didn't waste His energy refuting the devil's lie when I said, "She's just a fetus. It's not like she can actually *do* anything." He just continued to love me, saying, "Look at her!" with *delight* in His voice.

In contrast to God, I did the wrong thing in the embryo vision. I responded to Satan's lie. When he accused me, I literally turned toward him and asked to hear more. I said, "I'm bad?" I might as well have said, "Tell me more about what you think of me, Satan!" Thankfully I woke up before he could. God is merciful.

Do you see the contrast between the embryo and fetus visions? In the embryo vision Satan judged, accused, and condemned me, and I wanted to hear more. But in the fetus vision God didn't say I was bad, and He didn't say I was good. He didn't judge me at all. He just delighted in me. And I didn't understand why.

Another contrast between the two stories is the number of times I had to hear the messages in order to receive them. The devil told me, "You're bad," only one time before I received it. But God had to emphatically tell me, "Look at her!" at least five times before I received the truth.

What does that tell you about human nature? We receive judgment and condemnation a whole lot easier than we receive God's love. I think that's another reason we sometimes read Scripture but don't receive it on a deep level. I guess that's also why Paul said in Colossians 3:2 to set your mind on things above. He didn't say to debate and argue with the things below. Those things below are distractions that just stress you out and tempt you to rely on false comforters when you should rely on God.

The next time the devil tries to pull you aside and accuse you, don't fall for it. He's just trying to separate you from God, like a lion separates its prey from the rest of the herd for easier pickings. He knows that if he gets you to feel isolated, alone, and defective, you'll be less likely to discover your true identity and purpose.

Rather, turn *away* from the accuser and turn *toward* God. Focus on what is right, good, and true. Remember, at those times you *feel* alone (because the devil's lies cause you to hide from God in shame), you are never actually alone. "Neither height nor depth, nor anything else in all creation, will be able to separate us from the love of God that is in Christ Jesus our Lord" (Rom. 8:39).

Why Couldn't She Look at Me?

A long while after my fetus dream God gave me another epiphany about what He meant when He said, "Look at her!" God wanted me to actually make *eye contact* with my fetus self, so I could read and "feel" her with a deep level of understanding. I have a psychologist friend who calls that connection thing "attuning" to your patient.

Recall that during the vision, little Fetus Rita's back was turned to God and me. She couldn't bring herself to look at us. I think the reason was shame. The accuser previously had told her (when she was a little speck of an embryo) that she was bad, so she was hiding from God and me, just as Adam and Eve hid from God after eating the forbidden fruit.

I'm sure my saying, "She's just a fetus," didn't help to encourage her. She felt bad about herself to begin with, and I topped it off by broadcasting that she was unimportant because she couldn't actually "do" anything. Not only did Satan lie to her, but I did too!

As you can see, my attitude toward Fetus Rita (i.e., my attitude toward *my own self*) was part of the problem here. Obviously I needed to work on some things!

Sensing the need to reconnect with this lost part of myself, I chose to revisit Fetus Rita in my imagination, apologize to her, and try to coax her out of hiding. I told her (among other things), "Honey, I'm sorry for what I said. I also know what the devil told you, but I want you to know he is a liar. God is good and always tells the truth, and God and I both find you *delightful*."

As I continued to tell her the truth to refute the lies planted in her mind by the accuser, she eventually turned around to face me. Once she did, I could tell by looking at the expression on her face that she felt relieved, happy, and accepted. I didn't reject her anymore, and she didn't feel shame, so she didn't have to hide from me anymore. The lie had been replaced by truth: both God and I find her *delightful*.

If you think this is some kind of religious woo-woo, you're wrong. Secular psychiatrists and psychologists use this going-back-in-time technique. They get you to reframe past memories with more objective truth. They call it "reframing." Some even help you do "prenatal regressions," much like what I experienced on my own with my two visions.

The difference is, unlike secular psychologists, I am adamant about reframing past memories in line with God's truth, which is absolute. Any other so-called truth outside of Scripture is shifting sand. That's why I recommend that my patients see overtly Christian psychologists and psychiatrists if they have a choice.

Interestingly I am not alone among Christians in the belief that it's good to seek godly counseling for your "hurt inner child." Not long ago I learned that one of my back-pain patients, a licensed Christian psychologist, uses similar techniques with his clients. He has clients bring baby pictures of themselves to the sessions.

My patient said that, initially, the patients look at their baby pictures and see only negative things, but eventually, through counseling, they begin to see their child selves more positively, and their adult selves feel better too.

Can you relate to these stories? Does your inner child hide in shame, with your back turned to God and others (and even to yourself)? If so, hear me clearly. Turning your back on God only makes it harder for you to receive His healing truth. No matter how ashamed or vulnerable you feel, the better choice is to stop running, turn around, and face God. He is slow to anger and quick to forgive. Ask Him to forgive you and tell you the truth about who you are. It's scriptural!

Psalm 51:6 says it best, "Behold, You desire truth in the inner being; make me therefore to know wisdom in my inmost heart" (AMP). Maybe it's time for you to break out your old baby pictures and pray over them, just as my counselor-patient does with his clients. Ask God for understanding regarding the times in your life in which you suffered trauma. Those images may help you reconnect with the younger part of you that needs counseling. I walk you through that in more detail in the fifth part of the book.

You Can't Earn Peace Through Good Works

I know from personal experience that good works don't bring you emotional peace. Back in college I was a compulsive eater and very overweight. I used to think, "If only I could lose another twenty pounds, I'll finally feel that I'm skinny and attractive enough." I also tried to get good grades (at least in part) to optimize my worth.

Later in life after I became a doctor, I still felt anxiety and a never-ending compulsion to accomplish more and more. I became board-certified in a subspecialty, learned osteopathic manipulation, and even wrote books. Work was my drug, and each successive accomplishment was my next "high." Unfortunately, no matter how much I accomplished, the rush was short-lived. I still felt the anxiety on a day-to-day basis, and I couldn't put my finger on why.

The good news is my anxiety decreased abruptly and permanently when I started uncovering the lies that I believed about myself. In hindsight I realized that the anxiety was because, deep down, I thought I was "bad," and I thought I had to achieve in order to be good enough. Who could have known?

Many of my patients believe lies such as, "I'll never amount to anything," "I'm stupid," "I can't do it," etc. Some of them work themselves to the bone to show the world: "I'm not stupid; I'm smart! Just look at what I did!" "I can do it. See? I'm a worthwhile person, after all." Or they fill their homes with possessions, accumulating new cars, new expensive purses, and other items to fill that impossible-to-fill spiritual void.

Take it from me—trying to establish your significance through your good works brings only short-term satisfaction. In the long run it exhausts you and robs you of the energy that you could devote to more important things.

My middle-aged female patients are prime examples. They come to me in a state of absolute exhaustion, physical pain, and stress-related illness. They're perfectionists, overcommitted, dissatisfied, and they have low self-esteem. Many had abusive, alcoholic, perfectionist, and/ or judgmental, absent, or neglectful parents. And many are overweight and caught in the futile cycle of emotional eating, chronic dieting, and chronic pain.

I tell them, "I'm glad you do good things, but have you ever wondered if your motives are right? When people feel inadequate deep down, they sometimes respond by becoming overly busy. They're trying to 'works' their way into feeling good about themselves."

In some cases my patients' answers might surprise you: "I guess I felt like I had to do those things to be a good enough Christian."

I go on to tell my patients, "Have you heard of the acronym 'BUSY'? It stands for 'Being Under Satan's Yoke.'" No matter how hard you try, you can't erase your low self-esteem and loneliness with good works. Your inadequacies inevitably catch up with you.

I help these patients the same way I helped myself—by prayerfully and thoughtfully seeking God's help to uncover the lies that drive them into excessive busyness. Once they begin to see that they were overcompensating (filling their lives with activity to feel worthwhile), they're halfway home.

A Dream That Left Me Feeling Stupid

There I was, standing in front of my high school locker, feeling completely and totally frazzled because I didn't remember my locker combination. I was going to be late for class again, and I had to take a final examination that day. How could I be so stupid? You'd think that I'd have learned my combination by now, being that I was a high school senior.

I had no idea at the time that I was having a bad dream (that's right...not a vision, but a bona fide nighttime dream). I wasn't actually in high school anymore. In real life I was a forty-something-year-old board-certified medical subspecialist who graduated from high school twenty-five years prior.

In my medical residency I scored on average in the top 10 percent of all doctors across the country on national standardized in-service tests. That plus my Ivy League education should have convinced me that I was smart, but on some subconscious level I guess I didn't believe it. If I believed I was smart through every atom of my being, I wouldn't have had a dream in which I felt stupid.

It's just another example of how you can know information on the one hand (that you're not stupid) but feel differently on an emotional level. You can know the truth but not feel it. Knowing and feeling are two different things. As I said, they're stored in different compartments in your brain.

I didn't like having that dream, but it came in handy as a teaching tool when I counseled Bill, who had stress-induced back pain. As I manipulated Bill's back, I probed into what stressors he was experiencing. Ultimately it came out that he was under a lot of stress at work. That's not a surprise. Patients almost always say that work is their number one source of stress. It feels less personal and makes you feel less vulnerable to think, "I'm under a lot of pressure at work," rather than, "I feel worthless in general."

Bill eventually admitted to himself and me that he felt inferior to his work colleagues because he was the only one without a college degree. He said he felt stupid compared to them. I told him to not worry because even if he had the college degree, he'd probably *still* feel stupid at times.

I went on to tell Bill about my locker dream and about the conversations I had with two of my doctor friends—about how we became doctors to prove to ourselves that we weren't stupid. Now that we're middle-aged doctors, I guess we feel it's safe to admit that. We have the "I don't care what you think of me anymore" middle-aged confidence that I would have liked to have had in my twenties.

There. Does that make you feel better? At least three doctors battled the "I'm stupid" demons at times in their lives. It kind of makes you wonder how many other successful people feel the same way.

No matter how many degrees you hang on the wall, the accuser doesn't stop accusing you. So it really doesn't matter whether you went to college or not. He tells you you're stupid either way. And you know what? Neither smart nor good is important to God. As I said, He created us for relationship and fellowship, not functionality.

I Didn't See Fetus Rita Through God's Eyes

It didn't hit me until long after the vision I had of myself as a fetus that God had another reason for saying again and again, "Look at her." I had been looking at Fetus Rita but not *seeing* her as God sees her. I looked at her as if she didn't have real value because she was only an unborn fetus. But God wanted me to see myself as He saw me, not clouded by the lie that Satan had previously told me when I was a tiny little embryo.

As an unborn baby Fetus Rita could do no good works to earn God's love. All she could do was float around in the womb and just exist and grow. I believe that's why God picked the image of the totally dependent fetus to convey the message that He loves "just because," long before I actually did anything in life to win points with Him.

If you are the kind of person who measures your worth based on your works, please receive the right message. I know I said it before, but let me say it again because it's important: God doesn't love you because of what you do for Him. He loves you because, with or without your good works, you're His beloved, delightful child.

We Judge, but God Loves

The accuser wants you to judge yourself and other people because either way you lose. If you judge yourself as "good," pride takes you down. If you judge yourself as "bad," depression, low self-esteem, and anxiety take you down.

As a TV pastor once said in a sermon, "There's a ditch on both sides of the road." So turn away from the accuser and stop listening to him as he tries to get you to judge. Don't engage in conversation with him the way I mistakenly did in my embryo vision.

Instead turn toward God, who loves you and finds you delightful. Read His Word, and listen hard and try to understand what He is telling you. You may have to hear the same message five or even five hundred times before you get it, because it's easier to receive negative words than it is to receive positive words. So read this chapter at least five more times, receive the message, and refuse to give up!

ACTION POINT
Questions to Ask God in Prayer

✿ Lord, will You reveal if I have been judgmental toward myself, others, and/or You? If so, will You forgive me?

✿ Is there someone I need to forgive for teaching me to judge? If there is, I totally and completely forgive [name the person], with no expectation of apology or remediation.

✿ If I am having trouble hearing You, will You try speaking to me in a different and maybe more obvious way to get Your point across to me? Through what means can I best receive You, Lord?

✿ If I still can't hear You, is it because I'm up against a barrier that I've created? Is there a lie blocking me from hearing You? Or sin? Or unforgiveness? Or is there something else blocking me from hearing You? I'm sorry for [name whatever caused the barrier].

PART FOUR

TAKE CAPTIVE EVERY THOUGHT
How Right Thinking Leads to Right Actions

Chapter 10

TAKING CONTROL

I ENJOY WATCHING CHRISTIAN author Mike Murdock deliver his "Wisdom Teachings" from time to time. One of my favorites is "Wisdom Teaching #10: Your Focus Determines Your Feelings." Basically he says if you want to feel better and be happier, set your mind on positive thoughts. Think about your blessings in life rather than how people hurt you in the past.[1]

Let me give you a concrete example for how this works in my life. When I'm stressed out, I shift my thoughts to an upcoming trip to Hawaii my husband and I are planning. The vacation is to celebrate our twentieth wedding anniversary, but we also want to have a big, pull-out-all-the-stops family trip before our teenagers go off to college. We're going to visit Maui, Honolulu, and do the whole nine yards, God willing.

If I can paraphrase what Mike Murdock might say, just thinking about being in Honolulu is more calming than thinking about whatever else is bothering me. *Ahhhhh...Honolulu.* I can already feel the soft sand under my feet and the warm sunshine on my face. Even the word *Honolulu* is relaxing.

On second thought, speaking of sunshine on my face, I wonder what SPF sunscreen I'll need to pack for the family. And we'll need new swimsuits. Oh my gosh, I have no idea what to pack. I can feel the stress building.

It happened again. I was feeling good, thinking about Honolulu, but then my mind wandered to packing for the trip and I got anxious again. Do you see how it works? Your thoughts create feelings. Even individual words such as *Honolulu* create feelings!

If you don't already dwell on nice thoughts, let me give you an incentive to change your ways. Even scientific research shows that thinking negatively can make you hurt. A study published in 2010 in the journal *Arthritis Care and Research* showed that anger and sadness increase pain levels in women with or without the body-wide pain condition known as fibromyalgia.[2]

If you want to think and feel more of the thoughts that bring you peace and joy, not to mention experience less pain and improved health, read on. In this chapter I talk about how managing your thought life is a critical part of your long-term health maintenance plan.

The Atmosphere in Your Mind

"With God All Things Are Possible" (Matthew 19:26). That's what it says on the embellished, burnished gold wall hanging in my favorite exam room. The words on that plaque changed the spiritual atmosphere of our whole office building. Amazing healings—true miracles—have happened in my office, and I believe it's because my patients and I come into agreement over that scripture.

How about you? Do you believe that with God all things are possible? Do you believe that God can change you by revealing truth in your innermost places? If you don't, let me say it again: with God all things are possible! Write it on an index card and put it on your bathroom mirror. Say it out loud fifty times a day if that's what it takes.

Take Your Thoughts Captive

In 2 Corinthians 10:5 the apostle Paul told us to "demolish arguments and every pretension that sets itself up against the knowledge of God, and...take captive every thought to make it obedient to Christ."

Paul is basically saying, "*Pay attention!* Filter out thoughts that conflict with God's plan. Make yourself think the right way, and your right actions will follow naturally." I have found that doing so allows you to automatically feel better emotionally and makes you less likely to reach for false comforters.

You don't get apples from an orange tree, and you can't make good lifestyle choices flow out of bad thinking and emotions. Only Word-infused thoughts allow you to bear good fruit and become healthier in the flow of God's will for your life.

In practical terms this means if you feel an urge coming on to drink alcohol (or eat a sundae or buy your fiftieth purse), ask yourself, "Lord, what was I thinking about that triggered me to feel this way? Did something happen right before I became aware of that urge? What emotion might I be trying to avoid? Could those thoughts have tapped into a lie such as, 'I'm fat, ugly, stupid, or out of control'?"

It's a matter of self-discipline to police your thoughts and emotions in this way (and to continue to do so for the rest of your life). But it's a choice that reaps great rewards in the long run.

Straight Talk

As soon as I walked into the room to meet my new patient, Dale, he grumbled at me, angrily, "Doc, this is a waste of time. I already know you can't help me." He didn't even say hello!

When patients say I can't help them right off the bat, they're usually right. I can help only those patients who are actually *open* to receiving my help. Contrary to popular belief, not all patients who visit the doctor actually want their physical problems taken away. Their physical issues can serve as distractions from their emotional issues, which can sometimes feel more threatening to deal with. Pain and illness can definitely serve as crutches.

After evaluating Dale (or I should say, Old Grumpy) for another half hour, I decided he was right. He was one of those patients that I probably couldn't help. So, matching my communication style to his and not wanting to waste either his time or mine, I delivered his diagnosis point blank.

I said, "You've already seen the top surgeons, rheumatologists, orthopedists, neurologists, pain doctors, and OMM specialists in the country, and you're no better because your back is not your *real* problem. Your extreme negativity is your problem. I could practically feel it on you when I walked into the room. I just wasn't sure until I read through all your negative lab results and had a chance to examine you."

I went on to say, "Let me guess, you grew up in a very angry, negative, judgmental household. Now, in your adult life, you're surrounded by more of the same type of people. And you probably routinely say negative things like, 'I'm always going to hurt.' Am I right?"

You should have seen his jaw drop and the blood drain from his face when I confronted him. Dale didn't expect me to knock the chip off his shoulder and blame *him* for the other doctors' so-called failure to help him. If anything he was counting on adding another notch to his belt—me.

It was a pretty bold move to challenge him this way, I admit, but it worked to his advantage in the long run, which is all I wanted, deep down. I wasn't trying to be mean or coldhearted. I was actually just trying to defibrillate his heart with the truth before his brain figured out what hit him.

Besides, some patients love it when you rough them up. It builds your rapport with them in a sick, twisted, yet highly effective way that boggles my mind. Dale seemed to be one of those patients.

Sensing that Dale actually liked my approach, I continued to force-feed my best advice down his shell-shocked throat. I figured he wouldn't come back for a second visit, so this was my only chance to help him. It was like a Hail Mary in a football game you know you're going to lose anyway.

I said, "Each time your back pain flares up, Dale, I want you to stop and ask yourself, 'What was I thinking or talking about right before the pain hit me?' That subject matter probably was negative and either directly or indirectly triggered your pain to get worse."

By that point I knew that Dale was a Christian, and I even had his permission to talk about faith-related matters with him, so I went even farther out onto the limb and quoted Scripture. I said, "Replace those negative thoughts you rehearse with better thoughts like, Jeremiah 29:11, 'For I know the plans I have for you,' declares the LORD, 'plans to prosper you and not to harm you, plans to give you hope and a future.' Write that on a Post-it Note and put it wherever you'll see it most."

That's when the tables turned, and Dale left *me* shell-shocked. Instead of angrily storming out of my office, he actually asked me for the name of a good Christian counselor. Unfortunately I didn't know any *sadistic* Christian counselors, but by the grace of God, it all worked out in the end. Six months later Dale sent me a thank-you card saying he felt substantially better. It was one of those cards with an old-timey movie photo of Pollyanna on it. Had I known Dale had a sense of humor, I just might have and counseled him myself. (Oh my gosh! Did I just admit that in writing? Where's that backspace key?)

What Do You Ruminate on, Bessie?

Psychiatrists use the word *ruminate* to describe how people like Dale stew in self-defeating, negative thoughts. But do you know where the word comes from? It's a term used in animal science. When cows first swallow food, the food goes into the first part of their stomachs, the rumen. Later they spit the mish-mash back up into their mouths and continue to chew. This helps them more easily digest the grass. Because you're a human and not a cow, you weren't meant to ruminate.

One of my patients, Jada, ruminates on negative thoughts all the time. However, unlike Dale, whose back is normal, Jada really does have spinal issues. So I periodically give her injections at the hospital. But sadly she sabotages the results with her negative mind-set. She says things such as, "You can give me a shot, Doc, but I doubt it will help."

Part of the reason Jada hurts is that she has the unhealthy habit of taking responsibility for other people's problems. In a sense she carries them on her back. No kidding—her pain flares up when she watches the local news. If somebody else's house burns down, her back flares up. She's like a barometer for pain and suffering in Oklahoma City.

Thank God she didn't live here at the time of the bombing. She would probably have died from that extreme-stress-induced heart condition I told you about, Takotsubo cardiomyopathy. I'm not kidding, either.

Because I want to help her, anytime Jada says something negative around me, such as, "That shot won't help," I draw her attention to her negative statement and make her recant it. It's kind of a game actually. But it is also a polite way for me to broadcast, "When you come to my office, I will retrain you to cast off negativity and put on positivity. Not only is it better for *you* to do that, but it also protects the spiritual atmosphere of my office."

I do the same thing on my free online Christian weight-loss forum, www.EdensFreedomSisters.NING.com. If I didn't, the depressive Debbie Downers of the world would taint the atmosphere and discourage everybody else. Hey! It's my forum, and I have authority to police the posts to keep the site positive and encouraging.

The take-home message is this: the thoughts you ruminate on affect you and the people around you. Therefore, anytime you catch yourself thinking or saying something that's contrary to God's way of thinking, stop yourself, midsentence if you have to. Instead, recite the positive, healing truth found in Scripture. It can literally erase the spiritual effects of whatever negative thing you just said! In case you want examples of Scripture to use in your battle, visit Appendix B at the end of this book.

Filtering Out Negativity

"Lalalalalalalalaaaaa—I can't hear you!" Imagine yourself saying those words with your fingers in your ears. That's essentially what Pastor Steven Furtick said to do when people speak failure into your life. Jesus did it too!

Do you remember when Jesus was en route to the house of Jarius, the synagogue ruler, to save the little girl who was dying? He got sidetracked by the woman who touched the hem of His garment, hoping to be healed from her chronic bleeding. While Jesus was attending to her, the little girl died. Then men came from Jarius's house to meet Jesus, essentially saying, "Don't bother coming, because she's already dead."

On hearing of the little girl's death, Jesus *ignored* them. That's literally what Mark 5:36 says—"Ignoring what they said..." Jesus went to

Jarius's house anyway, taking only Peter, James, and John with Him to create the right atmosphere for healing.

Do people in your life speak negativity into your atmosphere? If so, pay attention to what you should ignore! Learn to scrutinize their statements and reject those that conflict with what God says about you and your situation. Surround yourself with people who speak good, right, kind, and true words into your atmosphere. Doing that will help to rectify and smooth your emotions so you can better succeed at weight control and everything else you set your mind to.

"Put On"

In Colossians 3:2 Paul says to "set your minds" on godly thoughts rather than on the thoughts of the world. Likewise in Colossians 3:12 he talks about "putting on" right behavior. That means it is something you must do intentionally, even if it doesn't feel natural.

Both of these elements, right thinking and right behavior, are choices that you make purposely. You don't suddenly fall into right thinking by accident, especially if you are like Dale and Jada and grew up in environments that taught you negativity and wrong thinking. Rather, right thinking and right behavior are learned habits. You reinforce them through repetition and self-discipline.

How about you? Are you ready to put on behavior that leads to better health? Are you ready to set your mind on Scripture and positivity? If so, let me give you some advice. After all, I've been going through my Romans 12:1–2 mental transformation on this subject for more than twenty-seven years.

Number one: give yourself time. You may want a life that is free of pain, illness, and all forms of hardship, and you may want that life immediately, but remember that Rome wasn't built in a day. It's more likely that your advancement toward overall health will occur in a step-wise fashion over time as you shed layer after layer of physical, emotional, and spiritual burdens.

Number two: don't expect to be perfect at controlling your thinking or your behavior right off the bat. If anything, expect to take one step backward for every two steps forward as you progress. If you catch yourself saying negative things, just recant your statements with scriptural truth, forget your mistake, and move on. Thankfully God's mercies are new every morning.

What Is the Flesh, Anyway?

I like the distinction a TV pastor made in a recent sermon. He said the flesh is not necessarily in your physical body. Though it's called "the flesh," for the most part it exists in your mind. It's a self-centered, self-satisfying way of thinking.

If you have the urge to eat a pound of chocolate, it's not because your stomach or your pancreas told you to do it. It's because your thoughts and emotions triggered your behavior to eat. Your fleshy desires originate in your mind.

Some people blame their literal flesh (their physical bodies) for their weight problems. They think there's something wrong with their hunger and fullness signals because they don't feel them. Or they look at their cottage cheese–dimpled bottom and say, "See. I don't know how to take care of myself."

Don't blame your dimpled cottage cheese bottom for your obesity. Your bottom didn't make you eat the doughnuts. Your fleshly mind made you eat the doughnuts that, in turn, made your bottom look like cottage cheese.

What on Earth Are You Saying?

You've heard the expression, "Sticks and stones may break my bones, but words can never hurt me." I wish that were true. Words can hurt. But they can also heal. Either way they're important and powerful and should not be taken for granted. (I'm actually talking to myself here because I have been known to be overly blunt at times, as you've probably already figured out.)

In terms of overcoming addictions, pain, and illness, be very careful to say positive, encouraging words that reinforce your success. Don't say, "Hello, my name is Suzie, and I have compulsive behavior problems." Say, "Hello, my name is Suzie, and by the grace of God, I overcame compulsive [name your vice here]."

Just as your thoughts influence your words and actions, your words also influence your thoughts, as it says in Proverbs 18:8: "The words of a gossip are like choice morsels; they go down to the inmost parts."

Your words are powerful. "The tongue has the power of life and death, and those who love it will eat its fruit" (Prov. 18:21). Use your weapon wisely.

Body Language

As I alluded to previously, I try to read between the lines of what patients say. Many times they unknowingly broadcast their root problems through their choice of words. For example, during treatment, my young patient Shane said, "My back feels confused, like it doesn't know which way to go." Basically Shane broadcasted, "*I* feel confused. *I* don't know which way to go, and I'm blaming it on my back because it's less of a psychological threat to do that."

Likewise if a patient says, "I feel a sharp, stabbing pain in my back," I might respond with, "Is there a situation in your life that causes you to feel emotionally stabbed in the back?" If a patient says, "My back feels locked up," I might say, "What situation in your life is locking you up or stifling you?" If a patient's feet hurt, I might ask, "Might you feel hesitant to take a particular step in your life for some reason?" If the patient's hand hurts, I might say, "Is there something you feel is more than you can handle?" If the issue is stomach pain from ulcers, I might say, "What's eating away at you?"

Be careful if you complain about constipation. You can guess what I might say. Now let me get back to Shane, whose back "felt confused." As I dialogued with him, I learned that he was at a crossroads in his career. He didn't know which career path to choose, and this stress and confusion manifested as back pain. He was literally carrying his emotional burden on his back. Moreover, once I met Shane's effeminate and flamboyant friends in the waiting room, I realized he was confused about more than just his back. He probably had a big conflict between his Christian faith and his perceived sexual orientation.

You can use this body language concept to your advantage. If you catch yourself saying, "My drinking is out of control," you probably mean, "I feel out of control in general." Or if you say, "I was bad today (in reference to eating)," then, you probably mean, "Today I feel like I am a *bad person*, and so I ate in a way that matches how I feel about myself."

What about you? What kind of language do you use to communicate your conflicts? What do you broadcast through your words or through your bodily symptoms? If you want to find out what emotions and beliefs underlie your tendency to reach for false comforters, then pay attention to the words you say and try to read between the lines to discover what you really mean.

An Emotional Load Tires the Physical Body

Do you feel tired all the time? Maybe you're emotionally burdened. In February 2012 a well-designed psychological research study showed that carrying secrets leads to the perception of physical fatigue. According to the study, "People who recalled, were preoccupied with, or suppressed an important secret estimated hills to be steeper, perceived distances to be farther, indicated that physical tasks would require more effort, and were less likely to help others with physical tasks."[3] For example, those who carried secrets of infidelity reported everyday tasks as requiring more energy to complete.

When the secrets were highly sensitive, such as in regard to infidelity or sexual orientation, subjects experienced the greatest degree of physical burden and/or fatigue. It was concluded, "Thus, as with physical burdens, secrets weigh people down."[4]

Emotion Contagion

Emotions are contagious. If you hang around with depressed or angry people, you may end up feeling more depressed or angry. That's not just my opinion or guess. Social psychology research in the areas of corporate negotiations, mob psychology, and employee-customer relations supports that this phenomenon is real.

People mimic the facial expressions, moods, and mannerisms of people around them. If somebody gives you a dirty look, you're inclined to return the dirty look. Or if a person smiles at you, you are inclined to smile back. Even though this can occur at the conscious level, most of the time you do this automatically and subconsciously, using mostly nonverbal communication.

I once heard Christian motivational speaker Lance Wallnau speak on this subject. He called the nonverbal communication "emotional Wi-Fi," which I thought was a pretty clever way of describing it. He said he uses that "Wi-Fi" term in secular circles, but when he talks with certain Christian groups (the more charismatic groups, I guess) he lets his hair down and talks about how demons might be involved.

Might there be "spirits of depression" or "spirits of anger" that jump off one person and onto you in spiritually oppressive atmospheres? I suppose it could happen. But if you want to stick to a purely psychological analysis, one possible explanation for how the emotions of other people affect you is a phenomenon that I mentioned in *The Eden Diet*: your actions affect your attitudes.

If you smile back at someone automatically (not even realizing you're doing it), then you become a tiny bit happier for having done so. Even if you don't feel happy at the moment you smiled, the act of smiling may boost your mood because your actions affect your attitudes. By acting a certain way, you convince yourself that you feel that way.

Unfortunately research suggests that happiness may be harder to catch than sadness. One recent study showed that each happy friend increased an individual's chances of personal happiness by 11 percent, while just one sad friend was needed to double an individual's chance of becoming unhappy.[5] *The take-home message should be pretty clear to you. Be careful whom you hang out with, lest their emotions rub off on you without you realizing it.*

Beautiful Thinking

Your thoughts and emotions make a difference in the image you project to others. Surely you've noticed that body weight isn't the only thing that determines beauty. I believe the degree of attractiveness people project (or don't project) has to do with how much fruit of the Spirit they feel. If people feel peace, love, joy, and all the other good things God promised, they beam with positive energy and are naturally more attractive.

On the other hand, if they feel fear, anger, worthlessness, and shame, they may literally repel other people, no matter how physically attractive they are under the doom and gloom. Without knowing it, you broadcast how you feel about yourself. You can be a physically attractive person that projects, "I'm unattractive," or you can be an overweight person that projects, "I'm beautiful." Either way, you're right. Your self-perceptions influence how others see you.

If you feel beautiful, you look beautiful. If you feel less beautiful, you look less beautiful. What you think and feel and believe about yourself actually manifests in your physical body. It also affects the way other people see you.

The good news I'm trying to convey to you is you can be even more attractive than you are right now by simply allowing God to change your mind. It's a lot cheaper and safer than plastic surgery.

The Central Goal

These strategies share a central goal—you can and must control your thoughts. Remember, this isn't just good advice—it's a mandate from Scripture: "We take captive every thought to make it obedient to Christ" (2 Cor. 10:5). In other words, pay attention!

Grab hold of the thoughts and emotions that cause you to reach for false comforters, and reject those thoughts that are based on lies and negativity. Dwell on what is right, good, and true, and be careful to say words that are right, good, and true as well. Let's talk more about practical ways to take control of your thought life so you can achieve the high degree of health God wants for you.

ACTION POINT
Questions to Ask God in Prayer

✡ Lord, do I dwell on negative or unhelpful thoughts?

✡ If so, did I learn this from a person or people, or was I born with this trait?

✡ Will You give me ways to overcome this tendency?

✡ Do I need to forgive anyone, including myself, for contributing to this mind-set? Lord, I totally and completely forgive [name the person or people] for being negative and/or influencing me to think the way they do. Will You forgive me as well? And will You help fill my mind with the thoughts that lead to peace, joy, love, and the other fruit of the Spirit?

Chapter 11

NO COMPARISONS

EVEN THOUGH I grew up in a geographical area that was highly Italian, I still felt different from the other kids. Part of the reason was I based my idea of "normal" on what I saw on TV. I used to watch shows such as *The Brady Bunch* and *The Partridge Family* and wonder why my family was so freakishly different.

Kids don't understand that TV isn't reality. Even the kids on TV aren't like the kids on TV. Child actors have armies of consultants to sculpt and manicure their TV images—not to mention psychiatrists who medicate them after their acting careers dwindle.

I even used to compare myself to cartoon characters when I was young! Believe it or not, I secretly wanted to be like Karen, the girl from *Frosty the Snowman*. For some reason she struck me as the ideal American girl, all cute and sweet with her blonde, poufy little ponytail and earmuffs.

Unfortunately in real life I was more like Lucy from *Peanuts*—an overbearing brunette girl with a penchant for amateur psychiatry. I know what you're thinking. I haven't changed a bit. Seriously, there's even a movie that perfectly illustrates how out-of-place I felt as a kid. The movie is *My Big Fat Greek Wedding*.

As a child the main character in this movie felt like a freak compared to the little blonde American girls in her class. She secretly longed to take Wonder Bread sandwiches to school as they did, but instead her mom packed the Greek dish moussaka. Her classmates called it "moose ka-ka."

From what I can tell, I'm not the only one this movie resonates with. My first-generation Mexican American, Middle Eastern American, and Asian American patients think the movie was written for them too!

The point is, television is a mirage, yet starting in our childhoods, TV and other media shape our concept of who we are compared to whom we should be. In this chapter I talk about how drawing comparisons leads to judgment and dissatisfaction, not to mention shame, guilt, and other emotions that could easily cause you to reach for false comforters. I hope that in the end you'll discover the truth that sets you free about these comparisons—and I'm not just talking about the fact that moussaka really is the better lunch.

Does Weight Loss Bring True Satisfaction?

On a subconscious level many people think, "I'll be happy and satisfied when I lose [fill in the blank number of] pounds." Yeah, right!

In a way it's like we chase mirages, thinking that if we can grab hold of that special thing we're desperate for, we'll finally feel satisfied. For some people the mirage is money. For others the mirage is having the perfect spouse or perfect kids. For still others the mirage is being thin and beautiful (notice that we lump the two together, as though the only way to be beautiful is to be thin).

Don't let this magical notion of weight loss be your mirage. Though weight loss will likely improve your health and self-esteem and maybe even extend your life, it won't solve all of your problems.

You'll never feel that you are "good enough" if you gained weight because Satan convinced you that you're bad, shameful, dirty, guilty, or ugly. If you harbor those lies in a thinner body, you'll *still* see yourself as bad, shameful, dirty, guilty, and ugly no matter how skinny you become. You'll always feel that you need to lose even more weight to finally feel good enough.

Or even if you do reach your goal weight, you'll start feeling bad about your car or your house or some other new mirage that you turn your attention to. "If only I had [a new car, bigger house, new dress], I'd finally be satisfied at that point."

Looking for Satisfaction

Eating food satisfies only the physical kind of hunger. It does little or nothing for emotional and spiritual hungers. If you're dissatisfied with your life on some deep level, no amount of chocolate feels like enough. If you lack an identity in Christ, no amount of melted cheese can fill that empty place. If you believe you're a bad person in general, ice cream and French fries just don't cut it. Not for long anyway.

In the short-term, eating those things takes your mind off of your deeper problem. But then, as you know, you end up feeling worse after you eat. You still feel empty and lost, but now you add the remorse from having been "bad" in terms of eating food you don't need.

In case you have fallen into the trap of looking to food for deeper satisfaction, God does not condemn you. God is merciful. He longs to help you with your *real* issues—the deep-down lies that make you feel unlovable or cause you to fear abandonment or rejection.

It's wonderful to feel the peace of God and to have the fruit of the Spirit. Those things truly satisfy emotionally in a way that food can't.

You Don't Want the False Comforter, Anyway

I once interviewed Dr. Marleen Williams, an eating disorders specialist, for my Eden Diet newsletter. During this interview she told me, "People don't necessarily want the food. They want how the food makes them feel." I was amazed that she could sum up so much of my own personal past experience in only two sentences.

In other words, if you feel bad about yourself (that you're fat, ugly, stupid, weak, etc.), you crave chocolate because it's smooth and creamy and sweet, just the way you don't feel at that moment. Consequently eating the chocolate momentarily brings you closer to how you wish you could feel.

That's why I dissuade people from focusing too much on which foods are right or wrong to eat. For many people, it's not really about the food; it's about what they expect from eating the food. They manipulate food to make themselves feel better emotionally when they feel ugly, stupid, anxious, depressed, angry, and so on. They expect food to satisfy them and return them to the "perfect" or ideal emotional state.

All this brings me to another important point. If you focus on what you lack rather than on what you have, you're going to feel dissatisfied more often and be more frequently tempted to eat food you're not actually hungry for. When you're dissatisfied, you're more likely to reach for a false comforter. So stop thinking about what you lack or what you're not and start thinking about all the blessings you have. Thank God for your blessings and for your identity in Christ!

I talk with my patients about "looking for the blessings" when I perform electrical nerve tests on them to detect nerve and muscle disorders. Usually I find simple things such as carpal tunnel syndrome (a pinched nerve at the wrist that makes the hand go numb, especially when doing your hair, driving, or putting on makeup). Carpal tunnel syndrome is easily corrected with a minor surgery if wrist splints and anti-inflammatory medicine don't work.

I tell my patients who fret over carpal tunnel, "Your condition is easily treatable, and it's not terminal, unlike the problems some other people I treat have. If you're going to compare yourself to others, don't compare yourself to 'normals.' Compare yourself to people who are dying of incurable disease. Then you'll feel blessed to have carpal tunnel syndrome instead of something worse."

Some of the most powerful ways the accuser manipulates your emotions is to get you to compare yourself to others, compare what you have to what they have, and to judge yourself and them in the process.

Don't do it! Don't compare yourself and don't judge, and you'll be less likely to experience emotional triggers. Thank God instead for your blessings (even if you have to try hard to find them), and you'll likely notice a dramatic shift in your attitude and emotions.

ACTION POINT
Questions to Ask God in Prayer

☼ Lord, have I hurt myself or others or You because of drawing comparisons? If so, I'm sorry. Will You forgive me?

☼ Lord, was I hurt because of someone else drawing comparisons against me?

☼ If so, is there someone I need to forgive? Lord, I totally and completely forgive [name the person or people, i.e., myself, You, others] for hurting me in this way.

☼ Will You help me learn to see myself and others as You see us rather than draw comparisons?

Chapter 12

HAVE NO FEAR!

WHEN I WAS five years old and it was time for bed, I didn't worry about monsters under the bed. I was more worried about the recurring polar bear nightmares. At least a half-dozen times I dreamed that a ferocious-looking white bear was plodding around in my backyard and trying to get me.

Thank goodness my favorite brown teddy bear comforted me in the middle of the night after those bad dreams. I clung to him any time I was scared.

Isn't it interesting the way my mind worked when I was a child? I was afraid of a polar bear in my nightmares. Yet when the dreams woke me, I sought comfort from my favorite stuffed teddy bear. You'd think I would have reached for some other species of stuffed animal, such as a unicorn or baby doll, rather than a stuffed version of the same type of creature that just scared me. Clearly the emotions of children are not always governed by logic.

Adults react to fear in equally illogical ways. We medicate ourselves with substances and behaviors that further destroy our health and our relationships. Or we subconsciously transform our emotions into headaches, back pain, rashes, and bowel problems because we can't handle feeling our anxiety directly.

If we were smarter, we'd just grab hold of teddy bears when we were afraid. At least doing that isn't unhealthy, dangerous, fattening, expensive, or illegal.

In this chapter I talk specifically about how fear manipulates you from your subconscious mind to cause you to experience physical pain and/or engage in unhealthy behavior. I do this so you can better recognize your own triggers for feeling fear.

When you realize what things scare you (e.g., feeling abandoned, vulnerable, overlooked, worthless, etc.), you can better isolate those fears and turn them over to God. In return you receive peace that is beyond understanding as well as lessened desire to reach for false comforters to medicate your fear.

What If There Really Is a Monster Under the Bed?

Danielle grew up with a very abusive, volatile, furniture-smashing, easy-to-enrage father. When she was young, she didn't have to worry about the monster under the bed or the polar bear in her backyard. She had to worry about the monster in the next room with the anti-social personality disorder.

"You're the problem," Daddy broadcasted to her when she was little. "It's your fault that I got mad and smashed the furniture. If you were good, none of this would have happened." OK, daddy dearest didn't directly *say* those things, but it was the message that seven-year-old Danielle inferred as she read between the lines of his violent outbursts.

Danielle's response was typical. When something bad happened in childhood, she automatically turned the spotlight onto herself and feared, "What role do I have in causing this? Am I guilty? Was I bad? Is what he did my fault?"

Many, many of my other patients think like Danielle. They're inclined to either blame themselves directly or take responsibility for the bad consequences of other people's choices, and consequently they're triggered to feel anxiety. "Oh, no! I must have done something bad again for this to happen."

Danielle also drew other conclusions in this situation with her father. Since she believed that her wrong actions caused her father's angry responses, she also believed that her right actions could cause him to stay calm.

In essence she convinced herself that her father's feelings and actions depended entirely on her. In a way she carried him on her back. If he was angry, it was her fault. If he was happy, it was because she did things right. She even concluded that her life depended on keeping him calm, because if he got too crazy, he might kill her.

Please learn from Danielle's story. If you're carrying responsibility for other people's emotions and behavior on your back, hear me clearly: It's not your fault that they [fill in the blank with their negative consequences]. For your own health it may be better for you to stop enabling others and release them to suffer the consequences of their bad choices. Otherwise you're allowing them to destroy you as well through the after-effects of your emotions.

Fear Can Cause Pain

Eventually Danielle became a middle-aged, overweight woman who came to me for back pain management. When she described her symptoms, she used the same words I've heard from a million other patients in her age group, "Doc, I'm just falling apart!" (Like the furniture, I guess.)

At first I looked for the usual physical sources of back pain, including alignment problems, spasms, disk problems, arthritis, and so forth. However, before long I realized that her biggest problem (even bigger than the physical part) was the way she handled the anxiety.

If Danielle was falling apart, it was because her "I constantly have to please and pacify people" anxiety drove her into frantic activity that mentally and physically wore her out. She was constantly either homeschooling her kids, chauffeuring them to ball games and practices, doing housework, cooking, volunteering at church, helping the neighbors, scrapbooking, or organizing neighborhood garage sales.

On top of that, even though she had a husband and kids to look after, she still carried responsibility for her father on her back as well as the self-imposed responsibility for keeping the peace in her extended, dysfunctional family. That was enough to wear anybody out.

Fear-Based Busyness Knows No Boundaries

From Danielle's example you can see that busyness can be driven by self-centered fears and anxiety. Perhaps you can even relate to her, no matter what your vocation is and regardless of whether or not you receive a paycheck for all your good works.

A different patient who comes to mind here is a stay-at-home dad. Jay is a man in his mid-thirties who about two years ago had neck surgery that failed to relieve his pain. The continued pain and the requirement for strong narcotic painkillers forced him to give up his truck driving job and stay home with the kids while his wife went off to work.

Within three minutes of meeting Jay, I had him pegged. Anxiety was compounding his physical pain problem. I should have called him "Mr. Fidget." He was clearly incapable of holding still for more than ten seconds in a row. He was a toe-tapping, pen-clicking, leg-bouncing, clearly restless and irritable kind of guy. For him to become disabled was probably a fate worse than death.

As a result of his deep-down unrest over being out of work (talk about a blow to the male ego), Jay threw himself into many good and worthwhile home-improvement projects for validation. However, since his motives weren't right, he continued to feel unrest, low self-esteem, and a sense of threatened masculinity over not receiving a paycheck. He also further aggravated his neck pain by doing projects such as painting the ceiling (which isn't wise if you just had neck surgery).

Are You Sure It's "Anger"?

In *Star Wars: Episode I—The Phantom Menace* Master Yoda said, "Fear leads to anger. Anger leads to hate. Hate leads to suffering." He also said, "Fear is the path to the dark side."[1] Jedi masters are pretty smart. Fear and anger are closely related.

When you feel afraid, you feel weak and vulnerable. Because you don't like feeling that weak, you perceive your fear as anger.

It's less of a threat to believe, "When you forgot my birthday, it made me mad," compared to, "When you forgot my birthday, it made me feel insignificant and vulnerable." The first statement puts you in a position of power, whereas the second puts you in a position of weakness.

In other words, if you think you feel angry, it's possible that you actually feel afraid. Maybe something led you to feel out of control, powerless, ridiculed, scorned, unrecognized, unappreciated, insignificant, humiliated, embarrassed, unimportant, invisible, abandoned, or unloved.

If you want to be less controlled by your emotions and feel less triggered to reach for false comforters, you must learn to identify your emotions correctly. And you must let go of your pride and be honest with yourself. If you think you're angry, ask, "Do I feel threatened in some way now?" The answer probably will be yes in some cases.

Fear, Pain, and Addiction

As a pain-management doctor I occasionally meet people who have been prescribed pain medicine for no obvious reason. Their imaging studies are negative, and there is no objective "proof" that they hurt. The vast majority of these people are not lying to get narcotics. Their pain feels very real. They just don't realize they're taking pain pills at least in part to medicate anxiety.

The German proverb says, "Fear makes the wolf seem bigger than he is," and I say anxiety makes your pain seem worse than it is.

When anxious people take pain pills, they not only experience relief from the painful nerve endings firing, but they also experience narcotic-induced relief of their anxiety. In turn the relieved anxiety is positive reinforcement for them to take more pills in the future. Some of them even become addicted to pills because of their underlying anxiety.

It's easy to see how patients' anxiety escalates in those cases when the cause of the pain goes undiagnosed. Especially if the imaging studies and tests are negative, patients bounce from doctor to doctor looking for answers and undergo even more expensive diagnostic tests that rack up bills and further compound stress.

They begin to think, "What if the doctors never figure out what's wrong with me and I die from this?" And, "I'm not only going to lose my job because my back hurts, but I'm also going to go bankrupt trying to pay off these bills."

Anxiety is a very real problem in the world of pain management. In fact, I believe it's a big reason why narcotic prescription abuse is on the rise. According to results from the 2010 National Survey on Drug Use and Health (NSDUH), an estimated 2.4 million Americans started using prescription drugs nonmedically that year. That amounts to about 6,600 new users every day![2]

If you struggle with pain plus anxiety, realize that God is a much better and more permanent solution to your anxiety. Before you take your pills, survey your emotions. If somebody "set you off" emotionally just before you noticed the physical pain, maybe you need something else besides a pain pill to calm you down. You probably need to pray and let God Himself soothe your emotions so you don't end up taking more medicine than you actually need.

(Perhaps it goes without saying, but if you think anxiety is leading you to overmedicate yourself, get specific instructions from your physician about how to decrease your use of narcotics.)

Tools for Conquering Fear

Recently before I was to give a national radio interview, I had to wait on the telephone line for a long time prior to the start of the show. During that time my heart started to race and pound, and I began to feel short of breath.

I recognized immediately that my physical response was due to anxiety. I've done radio interviews a bazillion times before and everything always went fine. Logically I knew I had nothing to worry about. But logic didn't help my heart rate slow down. My emotions were going berserk for no obvious reason.

Because I was so nervous, I couldn't think of the words to John 14:27 (the "do not let your hearts be troubled" scripture). All I could do was cover up the receiver and affirm the truth out loud, off the top of my head: "God is love. God dwells within me. Perfect love casts out fear. Therefore there is no room for fear in me. The fear is a lie."

Almost immediately after hearing my voice utter those words, the intensity and rate of my heartbeat went back to normal, and I was renewed with confidence that I would reach people for God. It turned out to be a great interview.

The take-home message is this: the next time you experience the physical state you associate with fear (the pounding heart, shortness of breath, impending doom, etc.), speak the truth out loud so you can hear it in your own voice.

Pseudo-Addiction

It's not just unwanted emotions and physical pain that drive people to their false comforters. It's also the *fear of feeling* the emotions and pain!

Did you get that? Let me repeat it. It's possible for you to actually fear "feeling."

I know because I had a very painful medical complication when my second child was born. My uterus and bladder ruptured after a failed "VBAC" (vaginal birth after Caesarian section—a procedure that is rarely done anymore now that we know it's bad).

By the grace of God both my son and I were fine in the long run. But at the time of his birth, we both nearly died.

After I was taken off the intravenous pain medicine pump on hospital day three, I was switched to oral pain pills. Let me tell you, when I knew my pain pills were being rationed, I kept my eye on that clock. As soon as the second hand hit the "twelve" on the fourth hour, I clicked the nurse's call button for my pain pill. "Click, click, click, click, click, click, click...." You get the idea (especially if you're a nurse).

Even though I was drugged, by the grace of God I was still coherent enough to receive an epiphany in the midst of my fervent call-button clicking. My *fear of feeling* the pain was worse than the pain itself, and it was leading me to overmedicate myself. In pain management we call this behavior "pseudo-addiction."

The truth is I wasn't a "drug-seeker." I've never in my life had a problem with narcotics. I was just scared. The pain was so horrific at times that I wanted to take the pill to prevent the pain from coming back. I was medicating my anxiety more than any actual pain by that point.

In Vivo Exposure

Just as I was afraid of feeling physical pain when I was in the hospital, some people are afraid of feeling negative emotions. Thus they reach for false comforters to avoid feeling anything at all. They drink alcohol, gamble, shop, or fall into other unhealthy behaviors that distract them.

In pain management we put people through "in vivo exposure" to desensitize them from their fears of physical pain. We teach them to keep moving (to an extent) even when they hurt. Otherwise they would fall into major depression as well as serious physical disability from lack of movement. If you don't move, you die. I like to think of this as being like tough love.

Because of this desensitization they see that nothing bad happens when they move around a little, their fear of feeling pain goes down, and their pain level automatically decreases too. That's because the fear and the pain feed off each other.

Perhaps you can trust God to help you with your own desensitization when it comes to experiencing your emotions. The better you can handle your emotions directly, the less inclined you may be to reach for false comforters. Maybe you should pray about finding a counselor to help you through that!

Perfect Love Casts Out Fear

Don't let your fear ruin your health by causing you to reach for false comforters. Pray for God's help so you can better identify the fear-based lies you believe about yourself, such as "It's my fault," "It's my responsibility," "I'm weak and vulnerable," etc. After you capture the lies the fear feeds on, allow God to replace those lies with His healing, loving, perfect, and calming truth.

ACTION POINT
Questions to Ask God in Prayer

✿ Lord, what is the root of my fear (what is my greatest fear)?

✿ Is there a lie buried in my beliefs about this fear? If so, what is the lie?

✿ And what truth do You want me to know that replaces the lie?

✿ At those times when I recognize fear, will You give me a symbolic weapon so I can fight the lies of the enemy? What is the weapon or symbol by which I can remember You and be strengthened? (I talk more about this in chapter 21.)

Chapter 13

POWER PLAYS

WHEN I WAS a toddler, I contracted a virus that caused my body temperature to spike up to 104 degrees. Because my body temperature rose rapidly, the high fever caused me to have a seizure. Though it happened when I was young, I was emotionally scarred by that scary event for quite a long time before God brought that memory to the surface and healed me.

There I was, little toddler Rita, lying on a gurney at the hospital after a seizure, being held down by a group of seemingly gigantic doctors in white coats who I thought were trying to kill me. You can imagine how petrified I was.

Intellectually, and in hindsight, I know those doctors were trying to help me. But at the time, through my confused, post-seizure, toddler perception and senses, it felt as if the people who were holding me down were trying to kill me.

Even though I had just had a seizure and was confused, I remember a little about the experience. I was terrified and physically combative, throwing a fit trying to get away from those enormous, scary people. Even now, more than forty years later, the image of the doctors' white coats and the feeling of vulnerability remain burned into my psyche.

In the years after that incident, on some subconscious level, I equated the image of the white coat with power and control. Never again would I allow myself to be held down by people in white coats against my will. If I had to be on one side or the other, I was going to be on the stronger side—the side that actually wore the coats.

I believe that irrational perception (that a coat could confer some kind of real power) is why I was intrigued by the world of medicine, even at an early age. The white coat represented safety and security, and I desperately wanted that.

Interestingly right after this hospitalization is when I started putting on weight.

Ding, ding, ding! Do you see the possible connection? If I could control nothing else in life, I still had power over the food I ate as a child. Eating helped me to feel better when I felt anxious and out of control in general.

I'm not the only doctor I know with a story like that. I have a doctor-friend who suffered a significant laceration to her head when she was five years old. Scalp wounds bleed a lot, and seeing the blood made her think she was going to die. She said that scalp laceration incident is why she felt compelled to become a doctor as well.

That makes me wonder how many other doctors out there became doctors because of their own childhood medical traumas. I imagine there are more of us than I realize.

How about you? Do you reach for false comforters when you feel anxious, out of control, or vulnerable? If so, for how long does your false comforter calm you down before you feel remorse? Alternatively how long is it before you have to suffer the consequences of using your false comforter?

In this chapter I help you capture the lies in your subconscious mind about power, control, anxiety, and false comforters. Once you grab hold of the lies that bog you down, you are in a better position to prayerfully release them to the Lord.

Darlene's Story

Darlene started gaining weight when she was about five years old. Later when she was eight years old, Darlene's father abandoned her family.

Though the two points in time don't seem obviously connected, to eight-year-old Darlene they were most certainly connected. She believed her dad stopped loving her, was embarrassed by her, and eventually abandoned her as a child *because* she gained weight. This knowledge made its way into Darlene's conscious awareness in her adult life when she was in Christian counseling and was no doubt inspired by God.

As you might guess, Darlene's fractured relationship with her dad poisoned subsequent relationships with men. She ended up marrying her career instead of a flesh-and-blood man.

Through her childhood experience Darlene learned that her weight could be used as a tool to keep people away in a broader sense. So that nobody else would abandon her, she overate to keep people away. Her weight gave her a layer of emotional protection, and it gave her a perception of having control in a dangerous situation. She rejected other people (especially men) before they had a chance to reject her.

Through the years Darlene succeeded in losing one hundred pounds on two separate occasions. However, each time she became smaller, she felt out of control. She couldn't control the flirtation with men. Losing weight caused her to feel vulnerable. It's no surprise that both times she regained all the weight and then some.

In a way I can relate to Darlene's story. I remember back in college overeating after freshman-year frat parties. If a young man stared at me in a drunken, lustful, stupor, it made me feel vulnerable, and I didn't like feeling vulnerable. In a sick, twisted way, it felt like it would have been safer to have a thick layer of fat to make me "undesirable."

Thanks to God, though, I learned better ways to keep people away. I no longer use my fat to speak for me. Now I am pretty good at "speaking" people away—like the time I spoke up to deflate the overbearing attorney who tried to intimidate me at my own office.

I had been treating this attorney's daughter, who was in a car wreck, and it came time to release her from active medical care. She was as recovered as she was ever going to be.

This attorney (who was extremely tall and quite a physically imposing figure) did not like that I was releasing his daughter. In my opinion he didn't want justice. He just wanted to milk the legal case for all it was worth. He wanted her to get more treatment so she could look good "on paper" when it came time for her settlement with the car insurance company. So this attorney physically invaded my personal space, towering over me and explaining in stern terms why I must leave the case open.

Boy, this guy was tall. If we were dogs instead of people, he would have looked like a Great Dane towering over little Dr. Rita, the Chihuahua.

This is where the Great Dane apparently underestimated the Chihuahua. Even though he got in my face, I didn't flinch, and I didn't take one step back. I just looked (way) up at him and in my yappy, barky way said, "Gee, it's making my neck hurt to look up at you from this close. Would you please take a few steps back?" *Bark, bark, bark!*

Chalk one up for the yappy little Chihuahua. Not only did the attorney step back, but he also apologized for standing too closely. His whole demeanor changed when I stood up for myself. It literally looked like he deflated. I closed his daughter's case that day, and he didn't fuss one bit more about it.

The Desire to Exert Control

JoAnn and Kyle graduated from the local university immediately prior to getting married in 1984. JoAnn had a bachelor's degree in philosophy and had a hard time finding a job after college, whereas Kyle, who had an engineering degree, quickly found a lucrative job in the oil and gas industry.

Though JoAnn was proud of her husband, in a small way she was also jealous. She too wanted to have a respectable career, authority, control, and admiration over her success. But at the same time she couldn't find an actual job that would allow her to use to her philosophy degree.

The three pregnancies that followed over the next five years of marriage led JoAnn to give up on her career goals entirely and become a stay-at-home mom. During that time she acquired a new habit of eating for emotional reasons, since she was stuck at home where all the food was. She felt unchallenged intellectually, frustrated, out of control, and sometimes depressed.

Perhaps JoAnn's lack of control over her career and eating habits was why she became so incredibly overcontrolling with her kids as they grew older. At least she could pressure her kids to act and look exactly the right way to bring her prestige. Their success in school, sports, and life became her success, and she drove them very, very hard to become everything she wasn't.

After JoAnn's kids grew up and left for college, her delicate equilibrium began to break down. She began to experience markedly increased anxiety, food binges, and weight gain, and she felt out of control. Her family doctor blamed it on menopause, but I think her problem was that she no longer had anyone at home to control and focus her attention on!

About this time JoAnn developed hip pain, which is why I met her. She came to me for treatment of the bursitis in the hip shortly after her forty-fifth birthday, and I gave her a steroid shot that helped her hip but unfortunately augmented the weight gain. She really didn't need that extra weight, considering that she was diabetic already.

Because of the intensified bingeing combined with the steroids, JoAnn reached nearly 220 pounds and hit rock bottom emotionally and physically during this time. Her diabetes was worse than ever, and she began to experience painful burning in the feet because of it.

JoAnn's primary physician suggested she undergo the lap-band procedure, which allowed her to trim down to 170 pounds over the next year. But she still had panic attacks and control issues. Because the lap-band procedure didn't address the root cause of her emotional instability (which I suspect was a deep-down lie from childhood, such as "I'm insignificant"), she ultimately regained all the weight and more.

As much as I want to tell you that JoAnn's weight-control story has a happy ending, I can't. I talked with her about letting go of her dieting crutch and her control issues, but she just wasn't ready or willing. Being a thinker and a person who intellectualized (recall that she was a philosophy major in college), she was too caught up in her head to actually feel and trust her hunger pangs. So after her second flare-up of hip pain got better, I let her go for a second time, without having treated the sense of deep-down insignificance that I saw as being the root cause of her weight gain and control issues.

Pride, Control, and Comparisons

First, let me define pride so we're on the same page. I didn't think I had much of a problem with pride until I looked up the definition. Then I was convicted. Big-time. Pride is all about how powerful you feel, how you perceive other people to treat you, whether you feel loved or respected, whether other people remember to worship you and follow your commands.

When your pride is hurt, it causes you to feel threatened, and feeling threatened, in turn, leads to fear (i.e., "anxiety"). In some cases fear turns to anger, because feeling angry is less of an emotional threat than feeling vulnerable. In turn the anger and anxiety lead you to say or do things that destroy relationships. Or those emotions compel you to medicate yourself with false comforters. You reach for the ice cream, drugs, cigarettes, beer, or name your poison; you head for the mall or the casino; or your physical stress-induced illness flares up. You have a flare-up of shingles, IBS, fibromyalgia, or you have a migraine. That's why author C. S. Lewis said that "pride leads to every other vice."[1]

It's best to remember the truth. No matter what your emotions tell you, you are not really all that powerful anyway (no offense). Neither are the people you measure yourself against in your endless comparisons. You are a flesh-and-blood, imperfect person, just like all those other people you compare yourself to.

When you feel powerless, realize that your false comforters do not make you more powerful, intelligent, appreciated, or respected. They only cause you to become overweight, drunk, financially destitute, emotionally miserable, and physically sick.

If you catch yourself feeling that your pride is hurt, or feeling out of control and vulnerable, *stop*, think, and pray before you act! Ask, "Is there something I'm afraid of? Do I feel insignificant? What prideful thought or fear is triggering me to fall into temptation? What lie do I believe, and what is God's truth in this situation?"

By asking these questions, you interrupt an automatic cycle:

deep-down lie → hurt pride → unwanted action

And you experience automatic emotional relief and fewer urges to seek out false comforters.

Your Flesh Does Not Control You

Some people put on handcuffs and offer themselves into bondage to different substances and habits. They believe they are slaves to their flesh—that they can't control themselves—when indeed they can control themselves but don't want to. Perhaps on some subconscious level, believing they are out of control relieves them of personal responsibility. They overindulge and then rationalize, "The devil made me do it."

In my mother's Italian dialect there's a colorful expression that when translated says, "The pregnant mother eats the egg, saying it's for the baby." Actually she's eating it because she wants it, just like you eat the sundae because you want it, not because you're "out of control."

Romans 6:16 says if you offer yourself to sin, you're a slave to sin. If you offer yourself to thoughts of sexual pleasure and adultery, you're a slave to those thoughts.

You have to stop saying things such as "The devil made me do it" and "I can't control myself." If you offer yourself to those thoughts, you will continue to believe those thoughts and you will continue to act on those thoughts. The truth is that you can do all things through Christ who strengthens you (Phil. 4:13) and "with God all things are possible" (Matt. 19:26).

You might as well be honest in those moments. Why don't you just say, "I could control myself and stop thinking about having sex with that person, but I don't want to"?

To break free from the lie that you're a slave to your flesh (in terms of weight control), you may consider purchasing the godly affirmations for weight-loss CD, titled *A Battle With the Flesh*, which is available at www.TheEdenDiet.com. In this CD I help you view your flesh as an impulsive little child so that you can (as a wise, mature adult) gain control over that child by loving him or her into submission.

Now allow me to recap the important points here. If your fears of being out of control manipulate you to reach for false comforters, take your thoughts captive and make them obedient to Jesus Christ. No matter what you would like to believe, only God is, was, and always will be the one in control.

ACTION POINT
Questions to Ask God in Prayer

✿ Lord, do I have control issues that hurt me, You, or other people?

✿ If I don't hear Your answer, Lord, is it because I am up against a barrier that I created? Might I believe a lie or be guilty of a sin, or do I need to address a problematic relationship first so I can hear You better?

✿ If I have set up a protective barrier and can't hear You, will You show me how to break through, get past, or overcome the barrier?

✿ Lord, if I am guilty of a sin that leads me to try to control, will You reveal the sin to me? I'm sorry I committed [fill in the blank] and hurt [fill in the blank]. And I extend forgiveness to [fill in the blank], who hurt me as well.

Chapter 14

REJECT PERFECTIONISM

CARLA IS MY fifty-seven-year-old business executive patient with perfectly sculpted hair, perfect teeth, perfect makeup, perfect nails, and perfectly matching clothes, shoes, and purse. She sees me for back pain that she developed after a car accident, and so far I have been able to help her feel 90 percent better.

Most people would consider that amount of pain relief to be a huge success, but not Carla. She continues to literally be consumed by her desire to feel 100 percent perfect and pain-free, even though she went into the car wreck at fifty-seven years of age with a lot of preexisting arthritis. Carla is a person who is used to being in total control in many areas of her life, so this lack of control over pain is literally driving her nuts.

Even though she made amazing progress in a short time, she continues to ask, "Why do I still hurt? Why? Why? Why?" Anyone could see that her emotional angst over the remaining pain is probably much worse than the actual pain she's trying to get rid of.

At her continued pleading, I told her why I thought she was continuing to suffer so much with her remaining pain. I pointed out that perfectionism might be adding to her stress level. Perfectionism and the strain it's causing her could actually be perpetuating her back spasms and blocking the effects of the OMM from fully taking hold.

She obviously didn't like my observation. When I suggested it, she replied, "How could I possibly be a perfectionist? I'm *not* perfect!

So I clarified, "I didn't say you *are* perfect. But based on the immaculate way you dress and the way you carry yourself, I can tell you want to be! I can only assume that you want your body to be 100 percent pain-free and perfect, and it's driving you nuts that it's not cooperating. That probably makes you feel out of control, which in turn adds to your stress level and perpetuates those few remaining muscle spasms."

You should have seen this woman's jaw hit the ground when I said that. She looked like I just saw her naked and without makeup.

I went on to explain, "There's a difference between being perfect and wanting to be perfect. It's the wanting to be perfect that causes all the problems."

I tried my best to deliver this information in such a way that reflected, "I understand, and it's OK." She could tell I was trying to help, so she received the information I gave her more graciously than I might have received it myself.

Though perhaps I was a little too blunt in my delivery (I had only twenty minutes allotted for her appointment and had to get to the point), my message to Carla was important: "As much as you want everything to be perfect, you're just going to have to relax and let God take care of it. Right now, as I physically manipulate your back, I feel like I'm playing tug-of-war with your emotional tension. I can't help you unless you relax and let me help you. "

In this chapter I lay a foundation for how perfectionism may relate to your problems, just as it relates to Carla's pain problem. I discuss how perfectionism may be rooted in low self-esteem and/or fear, and how it's rooted in lies that if left unchecked could lead you to reach for the wrong kind of comforters. Throughout the chapter I discuss how to overcome those lies by grabbing hold of the freeing truth of God.

More About Carla

Upon getting to know her better, I found out the true source of Carla's generalized perfectionism. It was the peculiar way in which she was raised. She wasn't just a perfectionist about her body and her appearance. She was raised to be a perfectionist in general.

Carla was adopted at the age of four by a wealthy couple and was their only child. Her adoptive father was generally absent, and her adoptive mother was her central caretaker.

Carla first began to experience excessive concerns about her appearance and her body at the age of seven. She recalled how her adoptive mother dressed her up in extremely frilly clothing, such as what you might find on a Victorian baby doll. Carla's hair was primped and curled and put up in ribbons. And she was taught perfect manners so she could be pleasing and courteous, as she was told a good little girl should be.

On the surface it doesn't sound so bad, right? At least her mom didn't neglect her.

Carla wished she had been neglected. If anything, being the only child, she was constantly hovered over and not always in a good way. More often that not she was scrutinized and judged.

She was horribly beaten if she got the slightest bit of dirt on those frilly dresses that she despised, and she was beaten if she didn't use perfect manners at all times. She felt like more of a showpiece than an actual daughter in that her acceptance into the family seemed conditional. If she didn't look and act perfect in the eyes of mommy dearest, she might be expelled from the family.

This perfectionism extended into her diet too. If she was given candy when she was a child, her parents immediately confiscated it, lest she get fat. She was never allowed to have any desserts, except for one or two bites of cake at occasional holidays or parties. However, she paid for it later by being put on a strict reducing diet for several days afterward, even though she wasn't overweight by any stretch of the imagination.

Even her aunt (mommy dearest's sister) was into perfection. One month before Carla's sixteenth birthday the aunt sent her a note saying, "Your sweet sixteen is next month. Don't gain an ounce so you can fit into your new dress!" Talk about a neurotic family. Can you think of a better way to make a teenage girl feel totally inadequate? I can't.

As a child Carla felt entirely unreal, just like one of those fragile, porcelain baby dolls that her mother dressed her like. She felt that if her looks, behavior, and eating weren't perfect, she might actually shatter.

"There must be something wrong with me, or Mother wouldn't have to try so hard to make me look pretty and act right. I must be bad or my real mom wouldn't have given up for adoption in the first place. I must be ugly deep down. I'm so ashamed. I suppose I have to try really, really hard to be as good and perfect as I can. I'll always try to look pretty and eat very little so I won't be fat and bad. Maybe I'll be good enough then."

With regard to how she ate, Carla learned as a young child to eat very little so she could stay slim, mostly because she was afraid of being taken back to the orphanage if she became fat. In other words, debilitating fear was the driving force in keeping her slim.

I imagine you wouldn't be surprised if I told you that Carla struggled with anorexia in her teenage and young adult years and then workaholism and perfectionism in later life. She was constantly working hard to try to be what deep down she thought she wasn't so she wouldn't be abandoned again.

Is Perfection Even Possible?

In a biblical sense it's not a sin to seek perfection. In fact, it seems that it could be good thing, if done for the right reasons. In 2 Corinthians 13:11 Paul said, "Finally, brothers, good-by. Aim for perfection, listen to my appeal, be of one mind, live in peace. And the God of love and peace will be with you." And in Matthew 19:21 Jesus said, "If you want to be perfect, go, sell your possessions and give to the poor, and you will have treasure in heaven."

Because Jesus and Paul said these things, we can conclude that it's theoretically possible to achieve perfection in a way that is pleasing to God.

I'm not a biblical scholar, but I think it's interesting that Jesus said in this translation, "If you want to be perfect" rather than, "You must be perfect," or even, "You can be perfect."

What if it never crossed your mind previously that you ought to try to be perfect? It sounds like Jesus wasn't necessarily campaigning for you to be perfect so you could barter for His love. He was just saying, "Look, if you have your heart set on being perfect, let Me tell you the right kinds of things to strive for."

Why would Jesus tell you it's possible to be perfect but not necessarily hammer away at you to try to do so? Because you're human and liable to be flawed, He knew you could potentially be hurt more than helped by striving for such lofty goals that most humans can't achieve anyway.

Perhaps one problem is that your idea of perfection is different from God's. The thing you strive for to make you feel more perfect (e.g., recognition, wealth, desirability, etc.) may not be what God sees as true perfection for you.

Are you conforming to the patterns of the world in terms of the kind of "perfection" you want? Or are you conforming to God's idea of what "perfection" is supposed to mean for your life?

According to Paul, in order to achieve perfection, you must rid yourself of *all* contaminants that affect the mind, body, and spirit. "Since we have these promises, dear friends, let us purify ourselves from everything that contaminates body and spirit, perfecting holiness out of reverence for God" (2 Cor. 7:1).

Did you catch that last part? Paul told you to correct yourself "out of reverence for God." Paul did not say, "Purify your body so you can be thin, beautiful, and finally get whatever it is that you think you're missing in life—a smoking hot date, more respect, more attention, more self-esteem." He also said to perfect yourself in "body and spirit," but usually when we diet we think only about the body and not at all about the spirit.

There is a difference between seeking perfection in a holy sense and being a perfectionist in a negative sense. As I see it, the difference appears to hinge on your motives. To strive to have a perfect, skinny body is not striving to achieve the character of God. It's striving to have what *you* think is perfect, according to the patterns of this world, not what *God* thinks is perfect (love, mercy, grace, and so on).

Should it be any wonder that your efforts to achieve this elusive goal of worldly perfection only get you into more trouble? Nothing good comes from trying to reach an unobtainable, unhealthy goal. Trying to do so just demoralizes you and makes you depressed.

Besides it's only through Jesus that can you attain true perfection in the eyes of God. "If perfection could have been attained through the Levitical priesthood (for on the basis of it the law was given to the people), why was there still need for another priest to come—one in the order of Melchizedek, not in the order of Aaron?" (Heb. 7:11).

Put still another way, if you could become perfect through your works, you wouldn't need Jesus. So I guess it's a good thing you're not perfect. Without the conflicts that led you to read this book, perhaps you wouldn't have a reason to draw closer to the Lord!

Why Do You Want to Be Perfect, Anyway?

Whether you strive for perfect eating, to be perfectly pain-free, or for promotions and financial wealth, what you're actually doing is trying to control the fundamental thought that scares you: "I am just not good enough unless things are perfect in my life." You're trying to "works" your way into security.

Do you see how this thought is rooted in fear? On a subconscious level Carla was afraid her adoptive family would abandon her if she didn't act right and look right. And this belief was reinforced by the fact that her biological mother truly did abandon her. Fear and insecurity drive perfectionism.

No matter what fearful thoughts underlie your desire to be perfect, remember the truth: "Fear of man will prove to be a snare, but whoever trusts in the LORD is kept safe" (Prov. 29:25).

Chasing Mirages and Perfect Patchwork People

Do you think having a certain "big thing" will finally make you happy? Maybe you want this season's latest Coach purse. Or maybe you want the new iPhone or iPad or season tickets to watch whichever sports team floats your boat.

At first, when you get the exact thing you long for, it makes you happy. But after a week or two (or maybe just an hour), you already long for *something else*. So you start looking around at bigger houses, better-looking spouses, nicer cars, or different careers. Or maybe you think, "If only I could lose another ten pounds, then I'll be happy again."

If you equate happiness with having some kind of "thing" or having "more" or being thinner, you won't stay happy for long. Basically you're just chasing mirages.

Don't equate happiness with being perfect or having it all. Stop thinking, "I'd like to have this person's cute figure, that one's hair, this one's bank account, so-and-so's clothes, his brains, her car, his house, her skills, that one's awesome vacations, and my neighbor's perfectly manicured lawn." This fictitious, perfect "patchwork person" you long to be, with the perfect body, perfect family, and perfect life, doesn't actually exist.

It's time to stop chasing mirages, longing for perfection, and trying to be a perfect patchwork person. Quit fantasizing about how perfect you would feel if you had a perfect family who lives in a perfect, squeaky-clean house. Your reality is that you, your family, your friends, and your coworkers are flawed, just like me, and it's OK. You can have peace and joy and excellent health anyway.

The Serenity Prayer

You probably have heard of the Serenity Prayer. It's commonly recited at Alcoholics Anonymous meetings and in various twelve-step programs to help people overcome addiction. But even if you don't drink alcohol or have an addiction, it's likely to still be applicable to whatever problem leads you to reach for false comforters.

> God, give us grace to accept with serenity
> the things that cannot be changed,
> courage to change the things

that should be changed,
and the wisdom to distinguish
the one from the other.
Living one day at a time,
enjoying one moment at a time,
accepting hardship as a pathway to peace,
taking, as Jesus did,
this sinful world as it is,
not as I would have it,
trusting that you will make all things right,
if I surrender to your will,
so that I may be reasonably happy in this life,
and supremely happy with you forever in the next.
Amen.[1]

—REINHOLD NIEBUHR

Whether you overeat, over-shop, over-clean, or take drugs, you're still doing the same thing as alcoholics. In order to deal with your imperfection and unwanted emotions, you feel the urge to compulsively *do* something (medicate yourself in some way) so you can escape.

The reason this prayer is so effective is it reminds you that: (1) God is in control and you're not, and (2) you don't have to be perfect to have a "reasonably" happy life. It takes a ton of pressure off of you. Basically, if I can paraphrase, this prayer says: "Whoa, buddy. Chill out. It's going to be OK. Things don't have to be perfect, and you don't have to be perfect. Instead, just shoot for 'reasonably happy.' In the meantime, just let go and let God."

Memorize this prayer and then recite it any time you catch yourself feeling driven by perfectionism. It may help reduce your anxiety as well as your compulsion to reach for false comforters.

ACTION POINT
Questions to Ask God in Prayer

☼ Lord, do I have a problem with perfectionism? If so, have I hurt myself, You, or others because of it? And will You forgive me? I am sorry I hurt [You, others, myself] because of perfectionism.

☼ Did someone else hurt me and contribute to my perfectionism? If so, I totally and completely release [name the person or people], with no expectation of apology or remediation.

☼ Lord, is there a root lie that led to my trying to be perfect? Did I believe something about myself, You, or others that is wrong?

☼ What is the truth that replaces the lie? If the lie relates to who I am, who do You say I am?

Chapter 15

MANAGING FAMILY STRIFE

As Leia's pain-management doctor I could both see and feel changes in her body when we talked about her family stressors. She, like many of my other patients, hiked up her shoulders to her ears and tightened the muscles of her neck and back when she talked about things that stressed her out—such as her family life when she was growing up.

Over the course of many visits I discovered that she inherited anxiety issues from her mom's bloodline and anger from her dad's bloodline. But were these traits genetics or learned, or could they have actually been passed down to her spiritually from her family tree? And what did that mean regarding what she might pass down to her kids?

I know it's possible to inherit spiritual burdens because Exodus 20:5 says, "You shall not bow down to them or worship them; for I, the Lord your God, am a jealous God, punishing the children for the sin of the fathers to the third and fourth generation of those who hate me."

If you want to break free from your family baggage that leads to spiritual and emotional bondage, read on. In this chapter I talk about the physical, emotional, and spiritual ways in which your family heritage can lead you to reach for false comforters. I also discuss how you can break free from oppression and experience greater health, peace, joy, and love through Christ.

Some Good News and Some Bad News

First, the good news: you are not necessarily destined to make the same mistakes your parents made or be plagued by the same problems. Your bloodline does not determine who you are. God determines who you are, and He says you're a "new creation" in Christ! (See 2 Corinthians 5:17.) By the grace of God you have free will (and through your reading of this book, the opportunity for emotional healing that your ancestors likely never had).

At a recent professional meeting I skipped out on a boring Sunday morning lecture to watch a TV church sermon. It was given by a female preacher from a local church. Her sermon was titled "You Have a King in You." She talked about the story of Josiah from 2 Chronicles 34-35. Josiah became king at eight years old. She said Josiah's father was evil but noted that his ancestor was Hezekiah, who was good and was in the lineage of David.

When Josiah was sixteen, he began to seek the God of his ancestors. At twenty years old he turned his country around, cleansing it of sin. He had a king inside of him, despite his less-than-optimal heritage.

This preacher's point was that you're not necessarily bound to carry on the sinful, dysfunctional, or sickly traditions of your bloodline. You have a king in you, Jesus Christ, just as Josiah had Hezekiah in him. So you can break free from the spiritual and emotional baggage in your family, grab hold of and thank God for the good qualities in your bloodline, and have a better life, just as Josiah did.

Now for the bad news: though awareness of your parents' mistakes helps you to avoid repeating them, you could still make an entirely different set of mistakes as you raise your own children! I learned this slightly humorous bit of wisdom from a patient many years ago. She said, "It's every parent's job to mess their kids up in an entirely different way from how their parents messed them up."

In our effort to be better parents than our own, we make other mistakes when we raise our own children. For example, the children of overcontrolling parents might raise their children in an overly permissive environment, and the children of overly permissive parents might become overly controlling.

No matter what lessons you learned from your own imperfect childhood, you can't be a perfect parent to your children because you can't be perfect. Only God, the Father in heaven, can be perfect and erase the mistakes that all of us make in parenting.

You Can't "Make" Other People Be Saved

Cathy was a sophomore at a local college. When I met her, she was dealing with several stressors: physical pain, academic stress, financial stress, self-esteem issues, and family strife.

After a few visits and a little probing on my part, I learned that Cathy's main stressor was her religion! She was the first one in her family to move to the United States from Korea, and she was the first person in her family to become a Christian. She was taking quite a bit of grief from her parents and brother and sister because of it. Most of them were Buddhist.

Perhaps you've lived long enough to realize that religion can be used as a weapon to destroy people's love for God. Some of us Christians beat up "nonbelievers" with our (sometimes distorted) views on religion, and we cause others to feel convicted instead of helping them to feel the fruit of the Spirit: love, peace, joy, etc. It's no wonder that some people turn away from Jesus when we present Him in a condemning way.

But Cathy insists she didn't do those things with her family. In fact, she said she never personally witnessed to anyone in her family. She never rejected them, so she has no idea about why they would reject her first!

She said the entire conversation about her newfound faith must have lasted about thirty seconds during her one and only trip back to Korea after leaving for college. She simply told her family that she had met a young Christian man and had started going to church with him. They were so shocked that they didn't say anything in response. The rejection came later, after she returned to the United States.

Why did her family reject her if she never beat them up with religion? Perhaps her family was upset just because she was choosing a different religion from theirs. Maybe they felt personally rejected. I'm just guessing.

The reason this whole subject came up is that Cathy came to see me for neck and shoulder pain. After I gave her a thorough examination and ordered an MRI of her neck, I found no physical cause for her neck pain, so I asked her about stress in her life, and this family strife is the subject that came up.

Figuring that God knew more about what she needed than I did, I asked her if I could pray with her about this stress. She said, "Yes!" So I put my hands on her shoulders and neck, and together we asked God to reveal the lie that the accuser wanted her to believe about this family situation. We also asked for God to reveal the truth.

Right there before me, even before I finished praying, she blurted out that she knew what the problem was. Apparently, she received a "word" from God immediately. She said, "They're *not my responsibility!*"

I admit I must have had a "what on earth are you talking about?" look on my face, because she said it again, but this time louder and with more certainty. "They're *not my responsibility!*"

It turns out it wasn't really the feelings of being rejected that bothered her, since she always felt different from her family. What bothered her is that she was burdened with feeling responsible for their salvation since they were her family and she was the first Christian in the family. She felt that she had somehow failed God by causing them to reject her before she witnessed to them!

With the revelation that they're not her responsibility, God reassured Cathy that she was not responsible for her family's salvation or lack of salvation. They have a choice, just as she had a choice. If they rejected her without her uttering a word to them about her faith, how could she help matters by actually saying anything? She couldn't. It was out of her hands, not her responsibility.

A prophet is sometimes unappreciated in his hometown. Sometimes people outside the family are needed to speak to the heart of your loved ones in need of salvation.

How about you? Do you carry the burden of a family member's salvation on your back? And does that cause you increased stress and heighten triggers to reach for false comforters? If so, take this information into the depths of your being: you cannot control other people's choices. You control only your own choices. So choose to pray for them and don't worry about the rest.

Adoption Lies

My patient Naomi was adopted at age four by a seemingly ideal older Christian couple, but they weren't as ideal as they appeared. They were having marital problems that were intensified by their last biological child leaving home. On some level they figured that if they adopted Naomi, it would knit their marriage back together.

Even as a young child Naomi realized that she was being used as a tool to hold together a shaky marriage. It made her feel very insecure and compounded her abandonment issues over having been given up in the first place. In her mind Naomi believed that her biological mother gave her up because she was bad. Thus she felt pressure to act right and knit her adoptive parents back together so they wouldn't get a divorce. That way she wouldn't be abandoned for a second time.

You can understand how these thoughts ("There's something wrong with me and that's why people abandon me. The only way I'm worthy is if I function as a tool. I'm not worthy of love unless I perform. It's my fault if they break up.") led her to be an overachiever later in life.

Another patient, Lauren, also internalized lies as a result of her adoption. Through a process called "inner healing," which I tell you more about in coming chapters, Lauren realized that there was a connection between the abandonment by her biological mother and her thirty-year struggle with irritable bowel syndrome (IBS).

As I spoke with her and worked on her with OMM, Lauren recalled an incident that occurred at age three when she had a potty-training accident. During this memory she recalled being scolded by her adoptive mother. Apparently as far back as when she was potty training, she worried that she would be given up yet again if she didn't do everything just right.

From her childhood until that day I treated her, Lauren expressed her anxiety through her bowels. When any event stressed her out, the IBS flared up. Interestingly, as soon as Lauren forgave both her natural and adoptive mothers at a deep, emotional level, her bowel symptoms nearly normalized.

Family Gatherings and Stress

I've been in private medical practice for fourteen years, but I've never, ever seen a more stressed-out bunch of patients than I did the day before Thanksgiving 2009. Every single patient said one of these three things that day: "We already have a houseful of guests," "We're leaving to be with a houseful," or "We have a houseful coming."

Isn't that funny? Thanksgiving is supposed to be a joyous time of family reunion, but the day before it ends up being the most stressful day of the year.

Why do we get more stressed out over holiday events with the family than we do about holiday events with friends?

One of my patients explained it this way: "You can pick your friends, but you can't pick your family. If old friends seriously wrong you, you tend to drift away from them and find new friends. But you can't divorce your family. You have to put up with their quirks, and I, for one, have gotten more and more tired of putting up with my family's quirks over the years."

I think the best solution for minimizing your holiday stress is to realize that others at those gatherings probably feel the same as you do. They probably have childhood baggage and pushable buttons too. In fact, you might even have added to their baggage and pushed a few of their buttons at times, since conflicts are rarely one-sided.

So realizing that you may be a part of the problem and that your family members were in the same boat you were back then, extend a little compassion and mercy. Let go of your bitterness, forgive those who hurt you, and act graciously without dwelling on who is right or wrong. And pray for the atmosphere of anxiety to be transformed into harmony, joy, and forgiveness. It's what Jesus would want you to do—for *your own* good as well as theirs.

Fear of Familial Abandonment or Rejection

If your parents divorced when you were young, or if you lost a parent to illness or tragedy, or if you were adopted, it's conceivable that you might have abandonment issues. If that's the case, later on in life you might secretly fear being abandoned all over again by your spouse. "When I turn forty, I'm probably going to be traded in for two twenties."

Or maybe you fear that your family will reject you if you stop engaging in dysfunctional behaviors with them. This would make sense if you are currently in an environment in which being over-weight, taking drugs, or drinking alcohol is the norm. Maybe you think your family will say, "Get lost, you snob. You think you're better than us now?"

Did you notice the common denominator between the different lies? They're fear-based. The accuser tells you that you're going to be abandoned if you stay dysfunctional, and he tells you that you're going to be abandoned if you lose the dysfunction. He basically tells you whatever he thinks you need to hear to get you to feel incapacitated when you're not actually.

No Such Thing as a Perfect Family

Even if you had the ideal childhood and experienced no physical, verbal, or sexual abuse, and your parents had no addictions or mental illness, you still didn't have a perfect childhood. If you think you did, you're delusional.

When a doctor says you're delusional, it's not just an opinion. It's a diagnosis.

How can I make such a bold statement without knowing you or your circumstances? Even if you were reared in the most perfect family ever, you were still part of an imperfect family. There are no perfect people, so that means there are no perfect parents or perfect families.

I had an interesting conversation with a patient on this subject. I suspected this particular woman (let's call her Jill) had an emotional basis to her mysterious pains, since all testing came back negative and none of the treatments I offered—not even OMM and trigger point injections—alleviated her unexplained pain.

So I asked Jill if we could explore how her childhood experiences might have influenced her current anxieties. I told her emotional stress can directly lead to pain that is "invisible" on imaging studies.

She said, "OK, but I'll just tell you right now, I had a perfect childhood. You won't find anything there."

On exploring things further, I found that to be far from the truth. Jill's mother was a heavy drinker, and though she never overtly abused her kids (she was a "happy" drunk), Jill grew up petrified that her mom would cause them all to die in a car crash. Jill used to even hide her mother's car keys and shoes so she couldn't drive anywhere when she was drunk. She loved her mother dearly, but she lived in constant fear that somebody—maybe all of them—would die because of her mom's drinking. Her life felt very out of control.

How did that cause Jill pain as an adult? Her back pain caused her to experience fear (fear of death, just like when she rode in the car with her mom out of control), and that feeling of being out of control made her pain seem worse. Though her initial back problem was fully corrected, she continued to have pain because her emotions kept her wound up and fearful.

Moreover, though Jill was one of several siblings, she was the only biological child her parents were able to have. Sometimes her adopted siblings would say things like, "How could *you* be unhappy? At least you weren't adopted!" My patient grew up feeling she had no right to ever feel sad because "at least she wasn't adopted." So she trained herself to never complain about her circumstances.

"Everything is perfect except for this darn back pain," she told me before we explored her childhood beliefs and attitudes. However, after we prayed together and asked God to reveal the source of her pain, she had the revelation that it's OK for her to feel unhappy now and then. She's allowed to experience negative emotions—*even though she wasn't adopted.*

The Influence of Family

Family experiences such as sibling rivalries and parent-child conflicts play a major role in influencing early childhood development. These early memories and events are often intermingled with shame, false guilt, fear, and even anger. Consequently we remain vulnerable when family members touch our exposed nerves later in life. Identifying our internalized false beliefs about ourselves from childhood can decrease the likelihood of reaching for false comforters in response to negative, family-induced emotions.

ACTION POINT
Questions to Ask God in Prayer

✿ Lord, do I have unresolved conflicts with family members, either living or deceased? If so, with whom?

✿ Will You create a new heart in me, so I actually *want* to forgive the involved parties for Your sake? Lord, I totally and completely forgive [name the person or people], with no expectation of apology or remediation.

✿ Lord, will You forgive me for hurting myself, others, and You through family conflict?

✿ Will You give me protective tools so I can interact with unhealthy family members without letting them push my buttons? If so, what do those tools look like? How do they work?

Chapter 16

FILTERING OUT LIES IN ADVERTISING

T HE ADVERTISERS KNOW my Achilles' heel," said Amy. "All they have to do is show images of melted chocolate, and in an instant I'm rummaging through the cabinets looking for sugar."

You've seen the commercials Amy is susceptible to. They show swirly, silky smooth-looking melted ribbons of luscious milk chocolate in the candy commercial. Or they show ribbons of chocolate being drizzled over the brownie ice cream sundae in the restaurant commercial.

Whether you realize it or not, advertisers manipulate your thoughts and your emotions through these ads. They not only make you want to taste the chocolate or cheese that you see on TV, they also practically make you want to *be* like the chocolate—smooth, creamy, pleasing, calm, accepted, and wanted.

Do you remember the Hershey's chocolate TV commercial that ran in 2008? It showed a Hershey's bar that melted into a series of shiny, chocolate-brown animated scenes, starting with a chocolate girl on a swing. The girl then melted and reappeared in a chocolate convertible with her boyfriend, which sped into the sunset being chased by chocolate bunny rabbits and chocolate butterflies.

At the end of the commercial the sultry-sounding female announcer said, "What makes a Hershey's bar pure? Pure simplicity. Pure happiness. Pure delicious."[1]

I say the whole thing is pure lies. The commercial was all about conjuring up emotions of satisfaction, fulfillment, being wanted and loved. It implied that you could feel warm and fuzzy if only you ate Hershey's chocolate.

Hear me now because I'm telling you the truth. No matter what the Hershey's company wants you to believe at the subconscious level, chocolate can't love you as God loves you. Chocolate is just food, and food is for the stomach. God is for your heart and soul.

If you think advertising is meant to educate, inform, or help you in some way, you are grossly misled. This is your wake-up call. Advertising is designed to *persuade* you and ultimately to get you to buy the products in question so the powers that be can make money off you.

In this chapter I introduce you to the various ways in which advertisers manipulate your emotions through slogans, jingles, and images, and trigger you to purchase their false comforters, which come in the form of food, cars, clothing, and other products and services.

Though the advertisers appeal to men in different ways (usually through their desire for sex and power), I confess I discuss mostly food advertising in this chapter. I'm an ex-compulsive eater so that's where my attention naturally lies. But you can apply the same principles to your area of weakness. It doesn't matter whether your problem is food, alcohol, sex, clothing, gambling, or some other issue, because the advertisers appeal to very common desires for acceptance, love, and power and control.

Besides, as I said in the introduction, since obesity has nearly reached epidemic proportions in our country, you could probably stand to lose a few pounds anyway. No offense.

Who Is Most Susceptible to Chocolately Smooth Advertising Lies?

Do you know whom this type of advertisement appeals to most strongly? It appeals to restrained eaters. In *The Eden Diet* I talked about restrained eaters. They're people who constantly try to exert control over what they eat, but then when their dietary restraint breaks down, they eat double or triple portions of what they perceive as forbidden foods. Basically restrained eaters are the same as chronic dieters.

Based on a study published in the scientific journal *Appetite* in 2009, restrained eaters prefer high-fat foods, and restrained eaters who were stressed particularly gravitated toward high-fat foods that are sweet.[2] Apparently the women in the study must have perceived that eating those sweet, high-fat foods calmed them down.

That's probably why chocolate and ice cream are so desirable to women. Women are more likely to be restrained eaters due to chronic dieting. If those women happen to feel stressed when they watch the chocolate advertisements, they are sitting ducks for being manipulated into eating chocolate (a high-fat, sweet treat that they perceive to calm them down).

What About Melted Cheese?

One of the funniest lines I heard a couple of years ago was spoken by the actress Nia Vardalos, the star of the movie *My Big Fat Greek Wedding*. When asked how she was able to lose so much weight, Vardalos said, "I broke up with cheese."[3]

Images of melted cheese on TV commercials mesmerize us as much as melted chocolate. You've seen the cheese melting over the steaming-hot hamburger patty and dripping off the nachos. You've also seen the ribbons of cheese being stretched between the pizza pie and the single slice that's being pulled away.

It has to be the high fat content of both the chocolate and the cheese that draws us. Fat makes food taste palatable. Plus, even though it takes longer to reach your bloodstream than do sugar and protein, fat causes much longer-lasting satiety. It sticks to your ribs and makes your warm physical fuzzies last longer than does sugar.

So the next time you see a commercial that shows melted cheese, or one where the devil (I mean the announcer) says, "Ahh... the power of cheese,"[4] remember what I said. Even though "cheeses" sounds like "Jesus," cheese is not lord over you. The only way cheese has power over you is if you behold the lie that it does.

Candy-Coated Deception

Unfortunately, because it was Saturday morning, my favorite weekday TV preachers weren't on. I had to watch regular TV while I walked on the treadmill. But thankfully what the devil meant for evil, God used for good. I saw a TV commercial that perfectly exemplified how the advertisers try to manipulate our emotions so we buy their products.

It was a Werther's candy commercial, and it showed moms and dads hugging their young children, causing the kids to look incredibly soothed, satisfied, and loved. The images alone evoked a strong sense of acceptance and love and made me feel like I was one of the children being hugged. The images also made me feel like a good mama (if only I gave my children Werther's candy, that is).

As though these intensely evocative images weren't enough to move me, the announcer actually came out and said two things that drove the message home: "There's just something about Werther's Caramel that makes a chocolate so smooth and creamy, you don't just taste it, you *feel* it."[5]

Busted! See? I told you commercials appeal to your emotions. As Dr. Marleen Williams, the eating disorders specialist, said, "It's not the food you want. It's how the food makes you feel."

The next time you mindlessly get up off your overstuffed seat looking for food during a TV commercial (when I say "overstuffed seat," I mean your couch not your bottom), stop and think about what motivated you. Do you feel like you're missing something, such as love and acceptance? If so, stop and pray to your heavenly Father instead of eating. He helps you feel like those children in the Werther's commercial—even without the candy.

When Are You Most Susceptible?

You are most susceptible to those advertising lies when you're physically hungry, namely when it has been several hours since your last meal. However, you're also susceptible when you're between hunger and fullness. As you might guess, you are the least susceptible immediately after a meal when you're already full.

A vast body of research on restrained eaters has borne this out over the years. Restrained eaters are most likely to cross the boundary line and eat forbidden foods when they are physically hungry. Conversely if they're already full when they are presented with tempting treats, they're less likely to break down and eat those treats. The Bible says the very same thing. According to Proverbs 27:7, "He who is full loathes honey, but to the hungry even what is bitter tastes sweet." When you're full, honey doesn't sound as appetizing as when you're hungry. That's why the advertisers bombard you with images of food at meal times and in the late evening hours. By bedtime you no longer feel the food in your stomach from dinner, so you're more easily influenced, especially by images of melted cheese and chocolate.

How do you avoid this sort of temptation? Maybe you can find different ways to unwind rather than watching television (which brainwashes you if you let it). Read Scripture or an inspirational book instead. Or make a late-night entry into your journal.

More Lies and Manipulation

Please forgive me if I sound snarky, but I am pretty tired of how the food advertisers try to manipulate us for money. First, let me pick on the Golden Corral restaurant chain, which adopted the slogan "Help yourself to happiness."[6] By suggesting that I can find happiness through its buffet line, the restaurant sends a subtle message that I must be unhappy. It also suggests that I need to fix that by eating. *Voilà!* They created a problem and then solved it for me in only four words. Slick.

"Help yourself to happiness" also feeds the consumer's fragile ego and offers hope. They're saying, "You can help *yourself* here! If you feel weak and insignificant, fix it by eating at our restaurant, where you have control and can feel better about yourself!"

Now, think about, "Come Hungry, Leave Happy,"[7] which is the slogan for International House of Pancakes, or IHOP. Their slogan basically says, "Happiness is the opposite of hunger. If you aren't happy, the solution is to eat pancakes. The profits will make *us* happy!"

How about Burger King's old slogan, "Have it your way,"[8] i.e., "You may not have control over many things in your pitiful, weak life, but when you come here, you get total control over your hamburger"? Fortunately they let *me* decide if I want ketchup on my burger. I wouldn't want the cashier to hold a gun to my head and force me to eat a burger with condiments I didn't like.

The irony is mind-boggling. These advertisers try to manipulate your thinking and your emotions so you buy their products, but at the same time they tell you that you're the one in control!

Since we're talking about manipulative advertising, let's not forget Mickey D's. A recent McDonald's slogan, shown on a billboard with a fancy coffee drink with whipped cream and drizzled chocolate, is this: "Instant Frown Remover."[9]

What does this advertisement really say? "Who needs Prozac, which takes six weeks to work? You can feel better instantly for only a couple bucks if you drink our fancy coffee. At least we're cheaper than Starbucks."

All things totaled, though, McDonald's most ridiculous slogan was the one they advertised in England in 2006. "*Make up your own mind.*"[10] That must be British humor, because I don't get it.

Advertising Lies That Suggest Food Has Power Over You

Previously I alluded to the American Dairy Association's slogan, "Ahh...the power of cheese," when I talked about how the commercials try to tantalize you with images of melted cheese. The idea is obviously to convince you that you are powerless to resist.

A Dunkin' Donuts advertisement is equally guilty. In one of its commercials children are being mesmerized by a tractor beam that pulls them toward the television. However, when one of the parents comes home with a dozen doughnuts, the kids immediately snap out of their TV trance, jump up from the couch, and run to the kitchen to grab for the doughnuts.[11] Thereafter, everyone in the family is laughing and smiling at one another with warm fuzzies as they eat the doughnuts, and all is well with this ideal little family.

The implication of the commercial is clear: if you want family time, or if you want to get your kids' attention away from the TV, feed them doughnuts.

What a crock. Kids who spend endless hours in front of the TV are already likely to be sedentary and obese, according to the statistics. Why make them more obese with doughnuts they probably weren't even hungry for to begin with? Does that really make you a good parent?

Other Advertising Lies

McDonald's once told you, "You deserve a break today."[12] In other words, "You've been working hard and deserve a break. You should eat."

Then KitKat candy bars took it a step further. Their slogan said it's "Break time. Anytime."[13] You don't even have to have done anything to justify taking a break. Eat just because you want to! At least the KitKat advertisers aren't "works-oriented" like McDonald's.

How about the advertising lies that equate food and acceptance? Olive Garden says, "When you're here, you're family."[14] They project the image of the lively Italians gathered around a dinner table, and you feel that you're part of the conversation and part of the family group. Doesn't that give you warm fuzzies and a feeling of belonging?

Too bad you have to stuff your face with breadsticks and pay money to get this nice feeling since your real-life family was probably dysfunctional in some way. As a person who grew up morbidly obese, let me personally attest that eating Italian food does *not* solve emotional problems.

And then there are the Pringles potato chip advertisements, "Once you pop, the fun don't stop."[15] If you're bored and feel you have no fun in life, just open the can of chips. It'll be an instant party—even if you eat alone! Do they really think my life is that lame?

They Lie to You
About What's "Healthy"

In a commercial for Special K cereal with chocolate chunks, a woman opened her freezer, saw a pint of chocolate ice cream, and heard the ice cream speak to her with a deep, sexy Barry White voice. The ice cream said, "You know you want me, baby."[16] However, the woman supposedly made the wise choice and elected to eat a big bowl of cereal, which the narrator suggested was a healthier snack than the ice cream.

What is wrong with this commercial? First, the large bowl of cereal the woman poured out was at least one-and-a-half to two full servings of cereal by my estimation. Add even if she were using skim milk, that bowl of cereal might have been at least 250 calories. Compare that to the 160 calories in one scoop of full-fat chocolate ice cream that the woman clearly would have preferred.

Next, ask yourself if the cereal is truly healthier than the ice cream. Do you think that cereal, which is made with chunks of chocolate, is better for you than the chocolate ice cream? If so, on what basis do you believe that? Do you believe it just because the announcer said so? Sucker.

On the basis of nutrition, that conclusion makes no sense. Neither one of those foods is more nutritious than the other.

Granted, there is probably a wider variety of vitamins in the cereal because the cereal companies probably added vitamin powder to the flakes. But what is the difference between that and swallowing a multivitamin each day while being able to eat the actual ice cream?

Now, factor in that the woman probably feels ripped off having eaten the so-called diet cereal, and, well, you know what she'll do later. She'll eventually pay herself back with some other sweet treat.

I'm not saying it's bad or wrong to eat the cereal. It might be a very satisfying breakfast or snack if you're hungry and that's the food you actually prefer. But make no mistake: it's not better for you than the ice cream, especially if you can retrain yourself to eat the ice cream in moderation (i.e., eat only one scoop) and take a multivitamin.

They Say You're in Control

The irony is overwhelming. Advertisers try to evoke emotions in you so you feel loved, satisfied, and powerful when you consume their products. However, they use language that manipulates you into believing you're the one in control! Don't fall for their tactics anymore, because you're being manipulated into eating more than you actually need, which in turn may cause you other kinds of misery down the line.

The next time a TV commercial assaults you with promises to change your life through some product or service, take your thoughts captive and also take my advice. Ask yourself these questions: What emotion does this message try to evoke in me? Does it try to make me feel powerful (as long as I buy this product)? And what is God's truth that refutes the lie?

After you answer these questions, you're in a position to accept or reject the message that's playing in your mind and act accordingly. You've followed the biblical wisdom of controlling your thoughts, a vital step in achieving control over the products and services you consume.

ACTION POINT
Questions to Ask God in Prayer

✿ Have I become dissatisfied with what You've given me because of advertising lies? If so, I'm sorry that my desires have hurt You, me, or others.

✿ Will You give me discerning eyes and ears so I can identify advertising lies in the future and deflect them?

✿ If I can't hear Your answers, Lord, is it because of a barrier that I created? Like sin that I haven't dealt with? Maybe sexual sin or some other sin? Or some other issue, such as unforgiveness? Or a lie that I believe about myself, You, or others?

✿ If it's the latter problem, what is the lie? And what is the relevant truth to replace it?

Chapter 17

CONFESSION AND REPENTANCE
SET YOU FREE

I AM IRRITATED BY the double standard in biblical times. Adulterous women were stoned to death with rocks that caused brain injuries and fractures, but adulterous men were only slapped on the wrist. I thought it took two to tango.

The priests even had a special test to check women for adultery. They put a kind of holy water in a clay jar, added dirt, and recited a predetermined "prayer." If women's bellies bloated and their thighs shriveled up after this ritual, it proved they had been unfaithful. (See Numbers 5:16–22.)

I imagine those priests were *very* careful to not get that water on their own skin during these rituals—for all we know, the special water might have worked on men too.

As a medical doctor I wish I had a diagnostic medical tool that worked like that magic detective water. It's hard to figure people out sometimes. Do they have a purely physical problem, or is their problem partly stress mediated?

"Mr. Smith, I'm going to sprinkle this diagnostic water over the area where your back hurts. If you puff up like a blowfish, your pain is from guilt due to sexual promiscuity rather than a bad disk, so we can skip the $1,200 MRI of your back. If the test comes back positive, I'll just throw this stone at your head and solve your back problem in a more cost-effective way."

If I tried this tactic, I don't think I'd have many repeat, bill-paying customers, though I'm sure I could drive down the cost of Medicare.

In the real world people like hearing that their problems are physical rather than a result of their own indiscretions. It's less psychologically threatening to blame physical things you can see on imaging. A "bad disk on the MRI" is easier to wrap your mind around than is "the consequence of mankind's sinful fall from grace."

However, because I care for you enough to confront you, in this chapter I explain how hidden sin, generational curses, and emotional baggage can in some cases contribute to physical illness, pain, unhealthy habits, and even premature death.

To make the unsavory sin pill easier to swallow, I try to talk about it in a way that isn't accusatory. See how delicate and tactful I am in my delivery? (Notice the humility.) OK, the truth is, I am trying to be tactful only so you don't pick up the stone and hurl it back at my own sinful head. I'm not perfect, either, as you can see from my false humility and bad writing. (In case you're wondering, those are the *only* things that make me imperfect.)

Spiritual Stressors

I work in the same town as the Federal Aviation Administration, the National Weather Service, and a major university. That means I have a number of scientifically minded patients, such as engineers, architects, and meteorologists. These patients are easy to work with because they readily understand how physical stress is transmitted through the different body parts. Toe pain could eventually cause knee, hip, or back pain (because toe pain causes you to walk funny and then your body compensates).

My patients also "get" how the mind and the spirit interact with the physical body. They understand physics, especially magnetic and electric fields, so it isn't a big jump for them to understand how "invisible" energy forces can cause bona fide physical effects. You understand this too, even if you never took physics in school. Just think of what happens when you try to put magnets together. The opposite poles attract and the like poles repel each other.

And think about how radio is transmitted. Invisible radio waves are transmitted through the air, generate an electric current in an antenna, and eventually cause the movement of air particles. The air then lands on your eardrum and triggers nerves in your inner ear to tell your brain you heard music. But you don't see the radio waves. The point is invisible forces, like stress, can have tangible, physical effects.

My science-oriented patients who are Christian can connect the dots even further, as they're used to having faith in a God they can't see. They acknowledge that invisible spiritual forces *such as unforgiveness and sin* can affect the physical body as well.

In Matthew 13:33 Jesus talks about physical manifestations of sin, but He does it by telling a story. He talks about yeast in dough, saying the yeast is like sin. You can't hide the presence of yeast if it's in dough. Eventually the yeast generates CO_2 gas, and the force of that gas expands the dough and makes it get big and fluffy.

Likewise, sin reverberates not only through your spirit but also through your body and mind, causing physical changes, accelerated wear and tear, and sometimes premature death. Don't let that happen to you, or if you do, at least wait until after you pay your doctor bills.

You Can Run but You Can't Hide

Even if you don't remember or recognize your sin, it could still be doing damage. According to Leviticus you can be burdened by sin that you forgot about, and even sin that belonged to your ancestors. You might even be running from a call that God placed on your life, as Jonah did.

A while back a TV pastor called a man up on the stage to share his testimony of a miraculous healing. For many months before the show was taped, the man experienced chest pain for which doctors found no cause. However, after listening to a sermon that pastor preached, the man experienced instantaneous supernatural healing.

At the exact moment of healing, God put this thought into the man's mind, "Stop running and go back into ministry!" After receiving these words, the man felt a rush of warmth fill his chest cavity, and the persistent chest pain vanished once and for all.

The man who received the healing was an associate pastor who left the ministry after a dispute with another minister. His spiritual conflict (having run away from God and the church) and the subsequent anger and bitterness were transformed into physical chest pain.

Do you want healing knowledge from God? Do you want to understand what makes you tick so you can overcome your unwanted behavior? Then repentance is a prerequisite. "If you turn at my reproof, behold, I will pour out my spirit to you; I will make my words known to you" (Prov. 1:23, ESV).

Detecting Spiritual Strife

Diagnosing spiritual issues, such as family curses, generational sin, demonic oppression, and so on, can be a lot fuzzier than diagnosing physical disease. At least with actual heart attacks you see EKG changes, blood chemistry alterations, and adjustments in heart contractility on echocardiograms. In contrast with spiritual disease, where you have no concrete proof. You have only suspicions and/or non-provable confirmations from God.

Sometimes knowing the patient's family and personal history gives good insight. With passage of time and the development of the doctor-patient relationship, the truth comes out about the patient's childhood, family dynamics, and repeating patterns of dysfunction. If certain patterns recur through generations, such as low socioeconomic status, incarceration, addictions, incest, abuse, diseases, and so on, I deduce that perhaps there's a generational curse in the patient's bloodline.

Or sometimes the patient tells me about past events that logically lend themselves to anger, unforgiveness, and guilt, so I can put two and two together. In other words, discerning spiritual oppression isn't always a matter of receiving woo-woo revelation knowledge directly from God about the patient, though it often happens that way. Sometimes it's just a matter of logic and deductive reasoning. If all the medical diagnostic tests are negative and the patient has a lot of pent-up negative emotions and unforgiveness or sin, I start thinking about potential spiritual causes.

When I discern that spiritual factors may be oppressing my patients,

I silently ask God to help me know what to do about it. His answers vary but have included, "Pray silently so the patient won't know," "Pray out loud so the patient can hear," "Use your authority to bind and/or cast out a demon," or, "Don't worry about it. I'll take care of it without you. Just keep your hands on the patient [or move your hands to this or that spot]."

Sometimes God answers in other ways. He says, "Do nothing. It's not the right time. I'll have you take care of this on a future visit." Or, "The patient doesn't want to change. Save your energy for the next patient."

If you think it's weird that a doctor believes in demons and generational curses, try to remember that I'm not just a doctor. I'm also Rita, a Christian, who believes the Bible is the inspired Word of God. The Bible has numerous examples of how spiritual factors such as demons and sin can lead to disease.

After Jesus cast out demons from epileptics, lepers, and the naked psychotic man in the cemetery, He said, "Go and sin no more" (KJV). To me that sounds like Jesus connected the dots between sin, demons, and disease. So you and I would be wise to do the same.

It Takes All Kinds, Not Just Faith Healers

I recently read a book on spiritual healing that was written by a preacher. His stance was that all physical and mental illness is rooted in sin, whether it's your personal sin or the sins of your ancestors, dating back to Adam and Eve's fall from grace. Ergo, in order to heal, you must identify and repent of your sin and the sin passed down through your bloodline. You must also forgive.

I like some of what the pastor said, including his explanation about the mechanism by which sin may be transformed into physical illness. He said sin causes emotional and spiritual stress. In response to this stress, hormonal and immunological changes ensue and cause wear and tear on the physical body that lead to illness.

But let me caution you so you don't come away from reading this book with misperceptions. I'm not sure the pastor and I see eye to eye on every point. Plus I think sensitive readers could misinterpret (or misapply) some of his points.

First, don't mistakenly conclude that "all" diseases and pains are necessarily rooted in sin, or that your disease is your or your family's fault. Hebrews 12:1 says to cast off sin *and* burdens. That means sins and burdens aren't the same thing.

In Andy's case a freak car malfunction led to his father's death and left five-year-old Andy with intense grief. Sin had nothing to do with it. It was through no fault of Andy's or his bloodline that his resultant emotional burden manifested as pain.

Second, don't accept condemnation for your illness. The pastor-author I am referring to does *not* condemn you. He seems to genuinely want to help. Unfortunately any kind of "Repent, ye sinner!" approach can lead some depressive individuals to condemn themselves. They twist his words and hear, "Repent, you idiot. You caused your cancer through your own badness." I know this because a few of my patients interpreted his message that way.

Third, don't conclude based on the pastor's (or my) patient examples that faith healing is the *only* "good" tool out there for healing illness. Deciding if a tool is "good" or "bad" depends to a large extent on the nature of the job to be done. Hammers work best on nails, not on screws and nuts.

On that "hammer" note let me point out a potential problem with the pastor's reasoning. He might possibly have fallen into the "if you give a person a hammer, the whole world looks like a nail" trap. He seems to believe that you should pray away your autoimmune disease, cancer, etc., rather than combine prayer with traditional medical treatment.

If he really does think that, I'd understand why (even though I think he's wrong). He counsels people who filter through the medical system without finding relief. His clients have a predominance of emotional and spiritual baggage, and because he applies the right tools to treat their underlying (emotional and spiritual) disease, they are more likely to get better in his hands rather than in doctors' hands.

In contrast doctors do better with patients who have actual *physical* disease as their primary problem.

I think there is an element of what statisticians call "sampling error" intertwined in this pastor's erroneous conclusion. It would be wrong for a faith healer or pastor to conclude that *everybody* should seek faith healing just because it works better *for some people* than traditional medicine. Likewise, it would be wrong for me to conclude that OMM works for *everybody* with back pain just because it works for a large percentage of the patient population that I see.

To drive this point home, let me go back to the tool analogy. Basically it's wrong to conclude that hammers are ineffective because they don't work on screws and nuts. Some screws and nuts are better served by psychologists and pastors than by doctors. Feel free to read between the lines of what I just said.

I think that's why God told me, "Rita, I want you to use *all* of the tools I gave you." He didn't say, "Rita, you should give up practicing medicine and just pray for your patients." Different clinicians have different gifts, and different patients need different venues for healing. My job is to be in sync with God's prompting so I can deliver what each unique screw or nut—I mean patient—needs, whether it is prayer, psychological counseling, diagnostic tests, shots, pills, procedures, or surgical referral.

Thankfully through the benefit of professional experience as well as wisdom and discernment, I have gotten better at identifying which of my patients need ancillary help and which will benefit more from a straight medical approach.

Don't Dwell on Past
Losses, Sins, and Mistakes

The angel told Lot to keep his eyes straight ahead and not look back at the burning city as he and his family fled. But Lot's wife disobeyed and looked back anyway. That's why God turned her into a pillar of salt. (See Genesis 19.)

Are you like Lot's wife and dwell on things from the past that you have lost? Maybe you look in the mirror and grieve over your wrinkles. I've caught myself doing that. On more than one occasion I've stretched my facial skin back over my ears to see what I'd look like after a facelift. But I didn't like the widened barracuda-lips look, so I decided to stick with good moisturizers (and non-magnifying, non-lighted mirrors).

Maybe instead of lamenting the loss of your youth, you lament a lost relationship, such as "the one that got away." Or maybe someone close to you died. In that case grief is understandable. But at some point you have to move on. God wants you to be happy again, and probably so would the person who died (if he or she truly loved you in return).

Maybe your problem is not lost youth, things, or people. Perhaps the problem is that you stew on past sins. Are you like the dog in Proverbs 26:11 that returned to its vomit? (I'm sorry to have used the words *stew* and *vomit* in the same paragraph. I hope you're not having stew for dinner.)

Instead of dwelling on your past sins and/or losses, look forward to the new things God wants to do in your life, as it says in Isaiah 43:19.

The Health Benefits of Confession

Truth be told, I don't like talking about how sin relates to our health. I always worry that people who tend toward depression and passivity are going to receive my words the wrong way—with self-condemnation and paralysis rather than conviction and commitment to change. But we can't avoid the subject because it feels uncomfortable to talk about it. As it says in Romans 3:23, "For all have sinned and come short of the glory of God." Thus the health and well-being of every one of us is at stake.

Hidden sin kills us from the inside out. It sabotages our emotions by causing guilt and shame, leads us into unhealthy stress-induced behaviors, and destroys our physical health too. "For the wages of sin is death, but the gift of God is eternal life through Christ Jesus our Lord" (Rom. 6:23).

In contrast, confession is good for our health: "Therefore confess your sins to each other and pray for each other so that you may be healed. The prayer of a righteous man is powerful and effective" (James 5:16). Confession immediately wipes our slates clean: "If we confess our sins, he is faithful and just and will forgive us our sins and purify us from all unrighteousness" (1 John 1:9).

Fence Posts and Weight Loss

Recently I heard this saying: "If you want a white fence post, you'll have to keep painting it white." Everyday life causes your little white fence post to get dirty. To keep it white, you either have to wash it or repaint it.

You probably already see how this "having to repaint your fence post" concept relates to your never-ending need to repent of your sins. Like countless other people I've spoken with through the years, including myself (whom I talk with regularly, often out loud), you may need to get back on the wagon over and over again throughout your life. It's a pain in the neck, but that's just how it is.

To move out of your past and into your future, take your thoughts captive, repent from your past sins, stop longing for things or people who no longer belong to you, reject condemnation for mistakes (because condemnation doesn't come from God), and set your mind on God's promises for your brighter, healthier future.

ACTION POINT
Questions to Ask God in Prayer

☼ Lord, is there an area of sin that I need to address? If it's sexual sin, is there an unhealthy spiritual connection that I created with that person or with those people (a soul tie)? I am sorry that I committed [name your sin here, sexual or otherwise]. Will You forgive me, Lord? In the case of sexual sin, in the name of Jesus, I break any and all soul ties with [name the person or people].

☼ If I am not aware of my areas of sin, is it because I set up some kind of protective barrier? If so, what is the root cause for that barrier? Is it another sin? Or a lie that I believe about You, me, or others? Or do I need to forgive You or someone else?

☼ If my problem isn't sin, is my problem fear or some other kind of emotion? If so, which emotion is bothering me? And what is the root of that emotion? Is there another sin or a lie or unforgiveness?

☼ Lord, if I still don't hear You, will You find another way to communicate with me? Or come to me despite my barrier?

Chapter 18

FORGIVENESS SETS *YOU* FREE

MY BACK PAIN patient Jason had a strained childhood to say the least. His father, Pete, suffered from bipolar disorder—a serious mental illness that involves periods of disorganized, manic, and sometimes psychotic thoughts, alternating with periods of deep depression. In addition to having bipolar disorder, Jason's father also struggled with addiction. He tended to abuse cocaine and alcohol, mostly during his depressed periods. In contrast, when he was sky high in mania, he actually *liked* how he felt, so he was less inclined to consume illegal street drugs.

Because Pete didn't reliably take his prescription psych medicine (he spent the money on street drugs instead), his wife found him impossible to live with and eventually filed for divorce, demanding custody of the children. Already in the throes of depression, the next step downward for Pete was suicide. Within two days of learning that his wife filed for divorce, he got drunk, snorted up his whole supply of cocaine, pulled out a gun, and blew his brains out.

There's more. Pete killed himself *right in front of his seven-year-old little boy.*

Just before he pulled the trigger, Pete tearfully apologized to Jason, "Son, I'm so sorry, but I can't go on like this anymore," as if his apology could save Jason from the ensuing years of despair.

Maybe you don't believe this story could be real. "Not even a mentally ill person would shoot his brains out in front of his kid."

Though I admit I changed a few details for my patient's privacy, the part about the suicide is true. My patient was in the room only a few feet from Daddy when it happened. He was close enough to have blood spattered on his face.

In this chapter I talk about how bitterness and unforgiveness, even bitterness directed toward God, can literally cause physical pain later in life. And I discuss ways in which you can move toward extending forgiveness, even after suffering childhood traumas or abuse as horrendous as Jason's.

Probing Deeper

Ironically when I first met Jason, I had no idea about his past. I didn't start probing into his childhood until after the MRI of his back showed only very low-level disk problems and the OMM and muscle relaxants failed to help. By then I was beginning to wonder about him anyway. The language he used to describe his back pain was a little too dramatic, considering the lack of physical abnormalities.

At first, Jason sincerely denied having significant childhood trauma. However, I could literally feel that *something* was wrong with him emotionally. It was like there was an elephant sitting in the room with us, and he couldn't see it. But that's what happens sometimes after you suffer a major trauma. You just block it out to protect yourself.

"You said the MRI showed a disk bulge, didn't you, Doc? Do you think I'm imagining this pain?" He was getting visibly ticked off as I asked about his childhood—maybe a little too ticked off. In itself, his overreaction was a clue.

"I didn't say you were imagining your pain. But I have a feeling that something besides that disk problem is adding to your stress. You know, stress can make your disk pain feel even worse."

I couldn't get Jason to open up about the childhood trauma thing, so I shifted gears. "OK, let's talk about spinal injections then." I was about to unleash my secret weapon.

"I can see you gained about thirty pounds since I've been treating you. At this rate if I have to give you an epidural, I'm going to have to use an extra-long spinal needle like this one." That's when I opened a drawer in the exam room and pulled out a spinal needle big enough to give the elephant in the room the epidural.

At the sight of that gigantic needle Jason became a little pale. That was the moment he suddenly remembered his father's suicide. He said, "OK, Doc. I didn't think this was relevant, but I just now remembered that my father killed himself right in front of me when I was seven."

"Thank you for telling me," I said, trying to hide that I was horrified. But I was really thinking, "You *just now* remembered that? How could you have forgotten it?"

Once the dam broke and Jason started talking about that tragedy, I pieced some things together by reading between the lines of what he said. It seemed that as a child he felt guilty, as though the suicide was his fault. It also seemed that he was angry with both his father and with God for letting the whole thing happen in the first place.

Lots of "Whys"

On the next visit Jason acknowledged that he felt somewhat better, even though I didn't actually touch him at the previous visit. He also thought about what I said—about how the suicide might be connected. He said he was beginning to wonder if it was true. You can't argue with non-contact pain relief. It's very convincing.

This visit was totally different from the others. Jason wasn't defensive anymore. And he didn't even talk about his back. For the most part he asked questions about what his faith had to do with his trauma. He apparently knew I was a Christian.

Almost tearfully, with a crack in his voice, he said, "I don't get why God would let something like that happen to a little boy."

I said, "I'm not a Bible expert, but I think God *had* to let it happen. Because God loves us, He gives us free will and the right to make our own choices, even if we end up making tragic, stupid mistakes that hurt other people. But don't forget, God is always there to pick up the pieces after we get hurt."

"So you blame *free will*?" He sounded sarcastic.

I answered, "No, that would be like blaming the gun. Your dad is the one who pulled the trigger. But lots of things contributed: the mental illness, his dysfunctional childhood, the cocaine use, and lots and lots of bad choices."

"Being that you're a doctor, I figured you'd say, 'You need to forgive your father because he was bipolar and didn't know what he was doing,'" Jason said with disgust in his voice. "I hated when people used to tell me that when I was a kid. It didn't help."

I replied, "I don't think your father deserves your forgiveness *more* just because he was mentally ill. What all of us *deserve* is to go to hell for our sins. But thankfully God forgives us because of grace, not because of what we deserve."

That's when Jason stopped looking angry and started looking ashamed, "I feel like a bad Christian for saying this, but I don't want to extend grace to him, and I don't want to forgive him. I want him to be punished."

"Hey! At least, you're honest," I said. "I used to feel that way about somebody I needed to forgive too. But Romans 12:19–20 says to leave the punishment up to God. I think it's because it's better for *us* to let God be the judge and jury. The spite just hurts us otherwise. "

"I never thought about that before, Doc. My wife and kids and I just became Christians about two months ago. All this 'forgiveness' stuff is still new to me."

"You're doing great. I don't mind answering a few questions. They're really good questions. I think you've been thinking about this longer than you realize."

"About thirty years, I guess."

"That's a long time. I imagine you're ready to feel better, right? If so, it's time to forgive your father. Matthew 6:14 says, For if you forgive others when they sin against you, your heavenly Father will also forgive you. You want God to forgive you of your sins, right?"

Jason was nodding.

I went on, "And you want your kids to forgive you for not being a perfect father? Then show them how to forgive. Be the role model your dad never was. Take the high road. Release your dad from any debt that you feel he owes you."

"I don't see how doing that makes a difference. My father is dead."

"Forgiveness doesn't help him. It helps you. And it helps your wife and kids, because when you feel better, it changes the atmosphere of your home."

"My wife and I have been fighting lately, so maybe you're right. I know *something* needs to change."

"Come on, Jason, let me help you. Repeat after me, 'Dad, I completely release you to Jesus, with no expectation of apology or understanding anything in return. You're not my concern anymore, Dad. Thank You, Jesus, for taking this burden off of me.'"

"I'm not ready, yet, Doc. Maybe later."

"No problem. Whenever you're ready."

About six weeks later at his follow-up appointment, Jason told me that God revealed something to him about his father. One morning while he was in that twilight stage between being asleep and being awake, Jason received three words from God, "He wasn't able."

Jason knew exactly what God meant. Pete lacked the ability to give Jason a sense of "normalcy" in childhood because between the dysfunctional childhood and the mental illness he didn't first have normalcy for himself. Nobody ever modeled "normalcy" for young Pete, so how was adult, mentally ill Pete supposed to model it for Jason?

The point is you can hold onto your anger and resentment as long as you choose, but you can't change the fact that *people can't give you what they don't possess*. Read that again: *People can't give you what they don't possess.*

I'm not in any way justifying the wrong behavior of those who hurt you in the past. I'm simply pointing out that everyone, including you and me, fall short in the eyes of God. If you want compassion and mercy, try to see others through the lens of compassion and mercy. Separate the sin from the sinner. I believe this and other ideas we talked about eventually helped Jason forgive his father and get rid of even more low back pain. It helped my patient Sandy too.

Sandy's "Aloof" Mother

Sandy initially had a hard time forgiving her adoptive mother for being emotionally detached. Her mom lost quite a few babies through miscarriage before she adopted Sandy, and that trauma left her emotionally shell-shocked. She was never able to come out of the fog to be fully present with Sandy and the other child she and her husband eventually adopted. Maybe she was afraid of losing them too.

Eventually Sandy was able to see her mother with compassion and forgive her with no expectation of an apology. In turn that definitely helped lessen Sandy's aches, pains, and anxiety. There was no real reconciliation, though, because Sandy's mother was still incapable of forming a close attachment with her kids. She was so detached that she couldn't even "read" Sandy to know there was a problem!

The physical distance between them didn't help. Sandy and her mother lived eight hundred miles apart. For financial reasons they saw each other only once a year and talked on the phone only once a month. Sandy never bothered to tell her mother where she fell short in the parenting department. It wouldn't have done any good. She just released her mother from the debt without telling her there was ever a problem. Talk about compassion and mercy!

Even more impressive was that Sandy apologized to her mother when, truly, she felt her mom deserved more blame. She said, "Gee, Mom. I just wanted you to know that I'm sorry if I ever hurt you." The mom said, "Huh? Oh, that's OK." That was it.

Mom didn't reciprocate with an apology, but Sandy didn't expect her to. She wasn't able. It didn't matter to Sandy, though. Sandy apologized for herself, not for her mom. Doing that helped her release one or two areas of guilt. You see, Sandy wasn't exactly perfect when she was a child either.

You don't have to always tell people when you forgive them. Sometimes they can't see past their own baggage or shortcomings to even understand what you're talking about anyway. At any rate, consider apologizing if you wronged someone else. Even if the other party refuses to accept your apology or is unable to receive it because he or she has barriers, apologize because it helps *you* feel better. It releases guilt, which can help you feel as good as when you extend forgiveness.

Pray for Your Enemies

This worked wonders for my patient Mark, a former US Postal Service worker. Mark carried resentment due to his career-ending, on-the-job right elbow and wrist injuries from slipping on the wet floor at work. Mark deeply resented several people who were involved in his worker's compensation claim, including his former boss and the coworker who indirectly caused his fall. He even resented the nameless, faceless US government as a whole for the injury.

All this unforgiveness made Mark feel miserable. No matter what kind of physical healing he achieved after his surgery, Mark still felt pain, partly because of his pent-up anger and unforgiveness. He also felt pain because of his downward spiral into depression during his first year off work. Thankfully Mark was a Christian and was open to praying for his enemies.

Mark admitted he was tempted to pray like this, "Lord, please help that adjustor moron to not botch up other cases like he did mine!" But he took the high road and, in my presence, forced himself to pray these words, "Lord, please bless that man. Give him good health, and help him to feel happiness and joy in his life. If he doesn't know You, put the right people in his life so he can come to know You. Maybe use me to reach him somehow."

The very moment Mark finished his prayer of forgiveness and looked up at me, I could tell by his facial expression that he had changed. He had tears in his eyes, and he looked relieved. He looked happier. He said he felt lighter and looser, and his wrist and elbow hurt less. People say those things when they shed emotional burdens.

Extending Forgiveness Is Better Than Retaining Spite

Recently I watched the *Hatfields & McCoys* miniseries on the History Channel. As I watched, I couldn't help but analyze the two main characters. Hatfield (Kevin Costner) deserted the Southern militia during the Civil War and left his neighbor, McCoy (Bill Paxton), to fight in his stead. Of the remaining soldiers, everybody from that Confederate troop died, except for McCoy.

When the war ended and McCoy returned home, his resentment toward Hatfield over the desertion grew and grew. Eventually McCoy's rage escalated the family feud further and led to the death of his sons, the insanity of his wife, his own alcoholism, and his accidentally setting himself and his house on fire while in a grief-driven, drunken stupor. His bitterness literally sent him to hell in burning flames.

I think McCoy either had survivor guilt, post-traumatic stress disorder, or both, due to the war. Furthermore I think McCoy unfairly funneled all of his anger and survivor guilt onto Hatfield, blaming him for more than his fair share. McCoy made Hatfield the "whipping boy" for everything that was wrong in his life.

In contrast, Hatfield tried early on to snuff out the dispute and let bygones be bygones. Unfortunately he couldn't keep his belligerent uncle from escalating the feud, and he couldn't quell McCoy's rage, so the conflict continued to grow, and Hatfield also lost many sons. At the end of the miniseries, at least Hatfield became a Christian. Compare that with McCoy, who claimed to be a Christian throughout but burned up in flames in the end due to unforgiveness.

Whereas unforgiveness and revenge compound your misery, extending forgiveness releases you from misery. As one of my patients said after forgiving her father, "It felt like the weight of a skyscraper was lifted off my shoulders." Which sounds better to you—the hellish consequences of bitterness or the uplifting freedom from extending forgiveness? Just remember what happened to Hatfield and McCoy in the end as you decide.

An Attitude of Gratitude

Recently I performed a nerve test on a patient who suffered great tragedy in her life. Some twenty-five years ago my patient's three-year-old daughter drowned. To make matters worse, her four-year-old son was at poolside when the three-year-old drowned, and ever since that time the boy blamed himself for his sister's death. During the son's teen years he began abusing drugs and eventually committed suicide over the accident.

It's a tragic story, but it has an important, positive lesson buried in it. The mom had carried otherwise unexplainable chest pain ever since her daughter's death, and as you might imagine, it got worse when her loss was compounded by her son's suicide. Eventually, as she proceeded through the normal grieving process, a change in the mom's attitude and thoughts allowed her chest pain to go away. Instead of continuing to think, "Why did God allow this tragedy?" she was finally able to forgive God for allowing her loss. She also learned to thank God for the short time she had with her children.

Almost instantaneously her attitude of gratitude and forgiveness literally healed her physical body. Isn't that encouraging? It means you have some degree of control over your physical pain. By adopting an attitude of not only forgiveness but also thankfulness toward God, you can live a healthier, more joyous, and pain-free life.

Love and Forgiveness

Do you believe God is love? It says so in 1 John 4:8. "Whoever does not love does not know God, because God is love." If you believe that God dwells in you, and you want even more of Him, you have to forgive those whom you hold grudges against.

Just as love gives us free will, love requires you to forgive. John 3:16 tells us that God so loved the world that He sent His only son to die for our sins. By sending Jesus to die on the cross, God created a bridge to connect Himself with mankind so He could forgive us and be reconciled with us. If God hadn't loved us so much, He wouldn't have made this kind of sacrifice. That's how important forgiveness is to God.

With regard to how many times it's right to forgive, "Jesus answered, 'I tell you, not seven times, but seventy-seven times'" (Matt. 18:22). This isn't to say that you must forgive those who hurt you in order for God to love you. If you choose unforgiveness, God loves you anyway. Just don't blame Him when you suffer the consequences of unforgiveness, such as stress, stress eating, obesity, physical pain, and illness.

ACTION POINT
Questions to Ask God in Prayer

✿ Lord, is there a person I need to forgive? If so, is that person You? Or is it me? Or someone else? Lord, I totally and completely forgive [fill in the blank] for [fill in the blank].

✿ Lord, where were You during the dark and difficult times in my life? Do I believe a lie about where You were in these situations? Or about how You are in general? If so, what is the lie? And will You accept my apology for believing You weren't there?

✿ If I cannot hear or find You in this situation, Lord, will You communicate with me in a different way so I can hear You?

✿ If the problem is a barrier on my end, will You reveal if I believe a lie or am guilty of sin or need to forgive someone so I can overcome the barrier? If not, will You reveal Yourself to me despite the barrier?

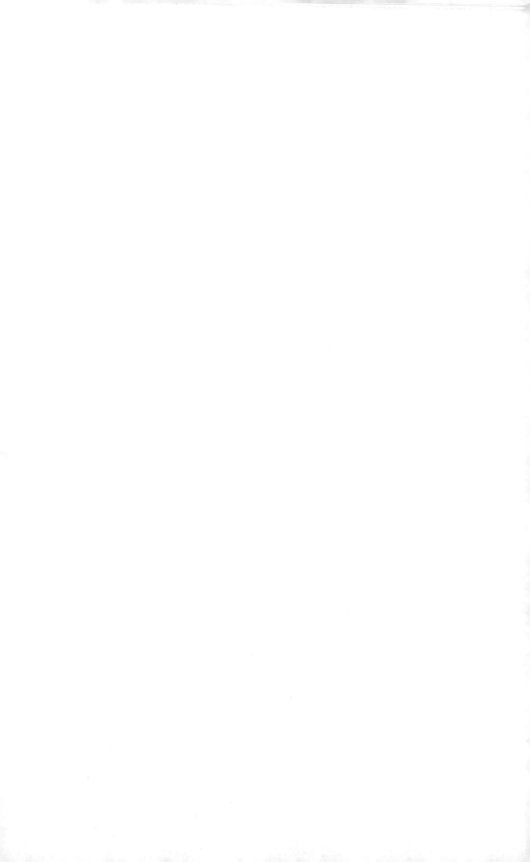

PART FIVE

HOPE IN YOUR FUTURE

Biblical Steps to Healing and Health

Chapter 19

INTRODUCTION TO INNER HEALING

AMANDA WAS A high-strung middle-aged woman whom I treated for shoulder pain, somewhat unsuccessfully until one day when she told me the real nature of her problem. For whatever reason she seemed to feel exasperated that day, and she blurted out, "It feels like my right arm is being pulled out of its socket, even when I'm lying down."

She went on to use other graphic words such as *ripping* and *tearing* to describe her pain, and the emotional overtones of those words got my attention. Knowing that her imaging studies were largely normal, I decided to probe into whether she suffered an emotionally meaningful trauma to that arm. Maybe it would connect the dots between her anxiety and her physical pain.

"Can you remember a time very early in your life, maybe a traumatic or stressful event, when you felt that same sort of pulling sensation on your arm?" I said, "Let God take you back to that, if you want to. You know I'm trying to help, so humor me and just relax and let go."

After a minute or so of silence, fear swept over her face and her whole countenance changed, "Oh, no. When I was three..."

When Amanda was three years old, she fell into hot asphalt that was being laid on the driveway of her new house in the suburbs. To try to get the tar off of her little body, her older brothers (ages eleven and thirteen) literally *pulled her by the right arm*, while she was kicking and screaming in fear, into the bathroom, where they stripped her down and scrubbed the tar off of her with gasoline-soaked rags.

As you might imagine, little three-year-old Amanda felt petrified.

She also felt ashamed and vulnerable due to her nakedness, even at her young age. Healing truth came to Little Amanda during the remainder of our visit when God assured her that He was with her the whole time and she would be OK. Still more healing truth came when she forgave all the parties involved.

If you are like Amanda and know God's truth intellectually (i.e., that God is in control of seemingly out-of-control situations) but still struggle with emotional issues such as anxiety, fear, and control issues, you might benefit from Christian counseling—specifically the type that helped Amanda. It's called inner healing.

In this chapter I tell you more about inner healing. I discuss variations of it that have worked for some of my patients. And I tell you about some of the pitfalls to watch out for, because not all inner healing ministers are equally qualified or have the appropriate finesse to use this tool.

What Happens During Inner Healing?

Inner healing is a prayer-based method of counseling that gets to the root cause of your emotional issues. It allows you to retrace your memories back to uncomfortable past events but with the full awareness and security that God is at your side during your healing journey. As you revisit relevant past situations during prayer, God Himself (not the counselor) literally places thoughts, visions, and/or ideas into your mind to draw your attention to events in which you might have internalized lies or misperceptions about yourself.

Different people receive knowledge from God differently, so God may speak to you in a multitude of different ways during an inner healing session. If you're a visual learner, God may give you an image that reminds you of a past event. Or God may simply give you a thought. Or He might cause you to feel an emotion such as fear that triggers the thought or image that takes you back in time. He might even cause you to perceive a certain smell that reminds you of a person or place from your past.

Or, as He did for Amanda (with the arm thing), God might give you a physical sensation that reminds you of a past event. God then reframes your perceptions about those events in the context of His healing truth and even helps you to extend forgiveness to the people who hurt you.

The benefits of inner healing can be astounding. It can reduce your depression, anxiety, anger, and other unwanted negative emotions, and markedly increase your sense of peace and confidence. After inner healing you may be more able to feel God's truth rather than just knowing it intellectually, and you may be less likely to reach for false comforters such as drugs, alcohol, and food when the people and situations around you rattle your cage.

In a way inner healing reminds me of a technique called "reframing," which I mentioned previously. But the main difference between secular psychological reframing and inner healing lies in what you consider to be absolute truth. Christian counselors use the Bible as a plumb line for truth, whereas secular psychologists use prevailing social norms (or should I say they use "shifting sand"?). That's why I prefer Christian counseling over secular counseling in the overwhelming majority of cases.

The Biblical Foundation for Inner Healing

Not only is it wise for you to seek inner healing, but it's also biblical. In Psalm 51:6 the psalmist said to God, "Surely you desire truth in the inner parts; you teach me wisdom in the inmost place." In case there's any doubt, your innermost places include the deep recesses of your mind, where you hide away painful and/or shameful false beliefs from your past. It's wise for you to open those places up to the healing light of God's truth, because He won't force His way in there to fix you without your permission, submission, and cooperation.

The most compelling scripture for inner healing is 1 Corinthians, where Paul talks about how the Spirit knows our thoughts better than we do.

> The Spirit searches all things, even the deep things of God. For who among men knows the thoughts of a man except

the man's spirit within him? In the same way no one knows the thoughts of God except the Spirit of God. We have not received the spirit of the world but the Spirit who is from God, that we may understand what God has freely given us. This is what we speak, not in words taught us by human wisdom but in words taught by the Spirit, expressing spiritual truths in spiritual words. The man without the Spirit does not accept the things that come from the Spirit of God, for they are foolishness to him, and he cannot understand them, because they are spiritually discerned. The spiritual man makes judgments about all things, but he himself is not subject to any man's judgment.

—1 CORINTHIANS 2:10-15

Words of Knowledge

Because this point is so important, allow me to emphasize it. Inner healing in its pure form discourages ministers from injecting their "words of knowledge" into your thinking. Rather ministers are merely supposed to assist you and pray with you as you receive truth from the Holy Spirit directly.

Perhaps I should back up and explain what I mean by "words of knowledge." Basically a "word" could be defined as a God-given insight about an event, problem, or situation in your life. It may come to you as a visual image, a literal word, a dream, a memory, a thought, a feeling, or a scripture that you suddenly recall. It could even come to you through another person, as words are sometimes given to one person to benefit another.

Here's the problem when people impose their words onto you: the information gets passed through *two* imperfect humans rather than just one. As Scripture tells us, we "see through a glass, darkly" (1 Cor. 13:12, KJV). Can you imagine trying to look through two consecutive blurry glasses? The image becomes even more distorted.

Do you remember the telephone game from elementary school? Your class sat in a big circle on the floor, and one kid whispered something into the ear of the kid beside him or her. Then that kid had to tell the next kid, and so forth. By the time the message got all the way around to the last kid, it was nothing like the message the first kid whispered.

That's the danger of relying on so-called words of knowledge from other people. Other people may not hear and understand God correctly in reference to your problem, they may not repeat the information to you in a way that you can receive it, and they may not deliver the message to you at the right time.

There can also be error on your end. You may not be prepared or able to hear or understand the message in the spirit that it was intended, or you may be flat-out unwilling to receive it.

It's even possible that friends, family, and fellow church members might deliver counterfeit words of knowledge to you. Whether they're consciously aware of it or not, they might be trying to manipulate you with the "word" so they can feel more in control, powerful, or important. That happened to me once. A minister gave me a word for self-serving reasons.

The obvious exceptions are when donkeys deliver prophecies to you (2 Pet. 2:16) or when the word involves specific information that only you and God know. Some words of knowledge are true and God-inspired after all.

The point is, when God puts a healing thought or word of knowledge into your mind directly, there is only one imperfect human involved (you). As a result, you're more likely to hear and resonate with the truth on a deep, personal level. You're also more likely to own the truth if it comes from the Counselor within you rather than through another imperfect person whose motives you may not trust.

I once attended a group inner healing weekend retreat at a very energetic, young church. Overall I'm glad I went because I wanted to see how inner healing worked in a group setting. Plus I met some awesome people, including ministers who were clearly anointed for healing.

But there was a fly in the ointment. *Every single participant* was presented with a "prophetic word of knowledge" at the end of the conference. I didn't think man could control the Holy Spirit to work on demand like that!

Seriously I think I know what was going on. These ministers were good-hearted people who really wanted to help. So out of their good intentions, they felt pressure to deliver a grand finale to the weekend course. That's why they "[spoke] visions from their own minds, not from the mouth of the Lord" (Jer. 23:16).

Don't misunderstand. I'm not throwing away the baby with the bathwater just because of that one drawback. This church was obviously an oasis of spiritual water in an otherwise dry community. I am merely saying you have to be careful about the information you receive from other people.

This reminds me of what my OMM mentor says in regard to new theories in his field. He says, "Eat the fish and throw away the bones." When you hear new ideas, pick out the good parts that you can use, and throw away the rest. That's exactly what I did after this weekend course.

A Fair and Balanced Perspective

A number of criticisms have emerged about inner healing. Some of them seem to bear merit, and others are probably discountable in my opinion. In this section I put forth my take on those objections, and I offer a biblical reminder that helps you put the whole picture in perspective.

One criticism about inner healing is that some people expect it to instantly fix or erase all their problems. I don't know where they get this belief. Inner healing does work extremely quickly to provide relief, and the relief is often significant and permanent. However, inner healing is unlikely to magically make anyone's life perfect.

I prefer to think of inner healing the same way I think of treating pain-management patients. One inner healing session might remove one or two dysfunctional layers from your onion. But there likely will still be other layers left over that need to be taken care of later, in other sessions. Still, taking off as little as one restrictive layer can translate into marked emotional relief, so it's worth it.

Another criticism is in regard to the qualifications of the ministers. Inner healers can be lay ministers in churches, or they can be licensed counselors, psychologists, and doctors. In other words, some inner healing ministers could be excellent and others could be downright dangerous based on disparities in their training—not to mention based on disparities in their natural gifts and talents.

Truth be told, this is actually my main area of concern too. Some inner healing ministers lack formal education in counseling, psychology, or ministry. Rather, they work as bank tellers and secretaries by day and, by night, are trained to become inner healers through homespun mom-and-pop programs within individual churches.

In my opinion, if the churches do not subject themselves to accreditation by an outside agency such as the International Society of Deliverance Ministers (ISDM), consider looking for a different inner healing venue. Just as our government needs checks and balances, inner healing ministries should have checks and balances too. Without outside policing, individual churches could easily veer off and "do their own thing," producing negligent or even cultish ministers.

That's why you must become educated about which ministries train their people in the most comprehensive ways and which ministries actually police their people with continued quality assurance assessments. Later in this chapter I tell you about two international ministries that are accepted by the ISDM and seem to meet the criteria that I insist on for my own patients. The ministries are called "Theophostic" and "Sozo."

Another supposed pitfall that I'd like to mention about inner healing is that inexperienced, improperly trained, or negligent ministers could theoretically insert false memories into your mind—i.e., make you think some kind of past abuse happened to you when it didn't really. Again, this is an offshoot of the problem I mentioned earlier in terms of inconsistent training and supervision.

If you seek help from a minister whose training is more rigorous, whose organization is affiliated with the ISDM, and who routinely gets continuing education and reevaluation and coaching from more experienced ministers, I believe this "memory planting" is unlikely to happen. However, if you go with a rogue, smaller, mom-and-pop ministry that lacks supervision and/or comprehensive training, "memory planting" could be more likely. As I said, whether inner healing ministers are good or bad for you depends on many variables.

With that being said, let's now shift gears and think about the financial costs involved. Despite the risks involved, once you crunch the numbers, you might decide to let inner healers unpeel your onion rather than PhD psychologists.

As you might imagine, it's more expensive to employ graduate-level psychologists and counselors instead of lay ministers. For example, a PhD Christian counselor that I sometimes utilize charges a flat rate of $275 per hour, regardless of the patient's financial situation. In contrast, a lay inner healing ministry that I utilize accepts offerings on a sliding scale. For as little as $50 you can get up to a three-hour session with *two* ministers. And both approaches are highly effective!

Forget about the cost difference, however, if you've experienced serious hurts, dangerous thoughts, and/or significant mental illness. In those situations you need bona fide doctors and possibly prescription medicine too.

Now that I've pointed out the potential pitfalls to inner healing, I beseech you to view this information from a God-centered perspective. Even though it's theoretically possible that individual churches could be lax in their inner healing quality assurance measures, I don't see ministers, pastors, and counselors with hearts for healing as being your primary enemies. The primary enemy is the one who tries to block your healing in the first place!

I'm talking about Satan, of course. He wants you to think your healing depends on the limitations of *people*, when it doesn't, really. Don't fall into this trap! Put your trust in God Himself, not in the people He works through. The Bible says it best in Psalm 78:21–22. "When the Lord heard them, he was furious; his fire broke out against Jacob and his wrath rose against Israel, for they did not believe in God or trust his deliverance" (NIV, 2011).

Put another way, if God makes a way for you to get high-quality inner healing through trained ministers, don't look your gift horse in the mouth. Trust in God, take your healing, and praise God's name for making things work out for your good.

Leave Your Agenda at Home

During your inner healing session, try to relax and have an attitude of submission to God, in the spirit of Romans 12:1. Be willing to receive any information God wants to give you, even if the path you're led down seems irrelevant or wrong. God knows what you need more than you do.

I remember one time during a session when God reminded me of something from my childhood. To my adult mind the event seemed trivial, and I thought I was being led down the wrong path. But to Little Rita (the seven-year-old part of me that actually experienced the trauma), the event was quite meaningful. Uncovering this layer was pivotal in freeing me from a layer of emotional bondage. Plus it laid the foundation for me to receive still greater healing at another inner healing session that occurred months later.

In other words, if you recall a major area in which you believe you need healing, such as if you were neglected, abandoned, abused, or hurt in some major way, don't assume your most painful memory will be the first layer God addresses. Perhaps you need to uncover less impactful layers first, as I did. Only God knows exactly what you need, when, how, and in what order. So relax, stop questioning Him, and let Him lead you.

Respected Resources for Inner Healing

Theophostic

One large and widely available Christian ministry for finding relief of lie-based emotional pain is called Theophostic Prayer Ministry (TPM). TPM is a prayer-based pastoral ministry that was founded with great success by Ed M. Smith, DMin, more than fifteen years ago.

It has grown into a worldwide ministry that has found its way into more than 160 countries by word of mouth.

The word *Theophostic* is made up of two New Testament Greek words that literally mean "God's light." *Theo* means "God," and *phos* means "light," like in the word *phosphorescent*. A TPM facilitator seeks to help the emotionally hurting person identify the lie-based core belief he or she holds at the memory experiential level. Once the person identifies his or her lie-based core belief, the facilitator encourages the person to connect with the presence of Jesus for His truth perspective.

However, TPM is not a "healing of memory" ministry. TPM does not teach that memory itself is the cause of the painful emotion. Rather, the pain is from the lie-based core beliefs that people hold in their memories. The lies can be eliminated and renewed with truth, but the memories per se should not be changed.

TPM is *not* in any way related to psychological counseling. A TPM facilitator should never diagnose, offer advice, give his or her opinion, provide steps of action, or direct or guide the ministry session in any fashion. Rather, the TPM website explains that if a ministry facilitator does anything during the ministry to move the session in any direction that he or she thinks it should go, then he or she is no longer doing Theophostic prayer.[1]

From the ministry's perspective, it's important to keep the session a "pure" Theophostic experience. Thus the minister should work from only TPM primary source material and not secondary sources based upon nonexperiential opinions.

The www.theophostic.com website has an abundance of information explaining more about the basic concepts. The website also includes firsthand testimonials and amazing results documented by doctoral-level researchers. Even though I give TPM a big thumbs-up for my patients, each person must check the material out for himself and ask his pastor or Christian counselor, psychologist, and/or personal physician if it's the right approach for him.

SOZO Ministry

Now let me shift gears and talk about a large and widely available inner healing ministry that helped me personally. It is called "Sozo." The word *sozo* means "to save, heal, and deliver." The ministry was founded by Pastor Dawna DeSilva of Bethel Church in Redding, California, and its aim is to help people find spiritual wholeness and peace.

Sozo practitioners help you shed spiritual barriers, find truth, repent from sin, and extend forgiveness. They do this primarily by helping you prayerfully *ask the right questions* to the Father, Son, and Holy Spirit during prayer. They call the question-based prayer experience a "Sozo" session.

If you liked the Action Point sections at the ends of the preceding chapters, you will probably love having a Sozo experience. Truth be told, in those Action Points I borrowed some of Sozo's very important concepts for getting through protective walls that block us from hearing or receiving truth from God.

In the world of osteopathic manual medicine, we call the physical walls that block movement and create pain "barriers." Thus, the concept of putting up walls that block us from hearing God resonated strongly with me. When I perform manual medicine on people, I position them up against their physical barriers of joint movement, and then I help them get past their barriers or walls so they can move more freely and with less pain. Why would it surprise me that this phenomenon happens in the spiritual realm too?

With that being said, keep in mind that what I presented in my book, including the questions in the Action Points, is nothing like an actual Sozo session. In Sozo sessions the questioning is much, much more effective than what can be presented in a book in a shotgun-type approach. But a true Sozo session takes longer too. A typical Sozo session is two to three hours. It also involves two fully accredited Sozo counselors helping you.

The material I present merely borrows from Sozo tools in a small way, and I mix what I drew from them with elements from my training in medicine, pain-management psychology, osteopathic manual medicine, psychiatry, and other healing disciplines. As I said before, the material I present is a mishmash of numerous strategies I've found helpful from a variety of healing disciplines. My methods are in no way, shape, or form a pure "Sozo."

As is the case with Theophostic, Sozo practitioners don't "psychoanalyze" you or offer their own prophetic interpretation of the meaning of your past experiences during a session. They just take you by the hand, lead you to God, and help you directly ask God the type of questions that bring you to a place of truth and healing.

Like Theophostic, Sozo is an international ministry with an excellent reputation for rigorous training, quality assurance, and policing of its practitioners. Both Theophostic and Sozo practitioners are basically told, "If you believe you get a word from God about the client during a session, keep it to yourself. Your job is to direct the client to God in prayer as he or she looks for answers, not to provide answers or interpret the meaning of past events."

In other words, "Don't get between God and the client. Just bring the two together and let God reveal the answers."

You can find certified Sozo practitioners across the United States (California, Michigan, Georgia, Massachusetts, Minnesota, Oregon, Texas, Delaware, the District of Columbia, and recently Oklahoma), as well as in Switzerland, Australia, the United Kingdom, Thailand, and other countries. If you want to become a Sozo minister or are interested in finding a Sozo minister in your area, visit www .bethelsozo.com. The ministry offers DVDs, seminars, and other educational material that will help you find what you're looking for.

Trading Faces

If you want to read an excellent book on Christian inner healing, read my friend Quinn Schipper's book *Trading Faces*. Pastor Schipper intrigues you with stories from his many years in inner healing ministry. He explains how inner healing can help those with histories of physical and sexual abuse, abandonment, and other traumas. Such experiences can result in suppressing emotionally charged painful memories and even fractionating into "alter identities" in order to survive. Though this phenomenon (splitting into alter identities) may occur in low levels in normally functioning individuals, it may occur at a pathological level in severe cases. In that case, we call it "dissociative identity disorder."

Pastor Schipper also addresses how to break free from generational curses and soul ties that indirectly trigger such things as anxiety, depression, and anger. At the time of this writing Pastor Schipper is no longer personally offering inner healing ministry sessions. However, his book is still an excellent resource for those who wish to understand inner healing from a Christian perspective. You can find *Trading Faces* via his website oikosnetwork.com or through Amazon.

Chapter 20

INNER HEALING IN MY
UNIQUE MEDICAL PRACTICE

I N MY NEARLY twenty years as a doctor I've accumulated a number
of therapeutic tools to help my patients experience pain relief.
These tools include oral medications, invasive injections, electrical
nerve testing, osteopathic manual medicine, asking the right questions (dialoguing), and, of course, prayer. But in all my years of practice I have never found a tool that is more amazing or works faster or
more permanently than inner healing.

Let me put things in perspective so you better understand how I
use inner healing in my practice. I don't want you to think I present
myself as a minister or psychiatrist, because I don't. Rather, I am a
medical doctor with a subspecialty board certification in pain management. And as such I am fully licensed to counsel my patients
regarding emotional issues.

It's just that periodically I meet patients who benefit more from
inner healing than from any other tool I offer. In those cases I set
my scientific knowledge aside and meet the patients where their problems lie—in the spiritual realm. In other words, with their permission,
I engage in this prayer-based technique for dialoguing, called "inner
healing." In this chapter I tell you how I incorporate inner healing
in my own medical practice in those situations when the Holy Spirit
orchestrates it.

Keep in mind that even though I describe what sounds like a rigid
"recipe" for what happens in the inner healing sessions, I am quite flex-
ible in following the lead of the Holy Spirit. Truly each session is different, just as each patient is different. Some sessions include many

elements I describe, and others include only one or two—or none—of the elements. And if things do progress, they don't necessarily follow any specific order. So don't think I apply a cookie-cutter approach when I don't.

Let me also point out that what I present is *not* inner healing in its pure form, and it's nothing like either Theophostic or Sozo, which I mentioned earlier. It's actually faster. Don't misunderstand—I didn't say it's better. Both are amazing. I just said my approach can be faster, and I believe I know why.

As a doctor I am licensed to touch patients during inner healing whereas ministers, counselors, and PhD psychologists can't. As you might guess, touching patients breaks down their barriers more quickly, so they tend to open up and spill their guts in a therapeutic way.

I also stand behind patients as I work on them with OMM. This helps on two accounts. First, they don't have to face me as they spill their guts. And second, my working on their backs serves as a distraction. They don't have to face their challenging memories head-on and with their full attention. Interesting stuff, huh?

Though it probably goes without saying, don't use the information I provide here as a basis for counseling yourself or others. You wouldn't take your own appendix out after reading a three-page description of how to perform an appendectomy, would you? I hope not. I present the information in this chapter only for you to understand the general principles that are involved. That way you can decide if you should seek this kind of help from trained professionals in your area.

Finally, please understand that my unique combination of treatment methods is not "endorsed" by any individual or organization of ministers, pastors, psychologists, or pain-management doctors, and it's not typical of my medical specialty. What I write merely represents the uniquely integrated point of view of one clinician-healer—*me*.

Who Receives Inner Healing?

It's not up to me to decide who receives inner healing. I never schedule patients for it, because the way I look at it, I don't control the Holy

Spirit. If you want to tell Him what to do, go ahead and try, but I'm out. God decides ahead of time which patients are going to receive inner healing, and He perfectly orchestrates my day to allow it. Just about every time I am led toward an inner healing approach, other patients don't show or cancel, inadvertently making time in my schedule for the patient in need.

Occasionally I have patients who schedule appointments, hoping for inner healing. Sometimes they even come from far away expecting it. But it doesn't work that way. Sometimes people come to my medical office expecting inner healing and leave finding what they really needed was a little OMM and a steroid shot.

As I said, the Holy Spirit is in charge of who receives inner healing. I'm not. I just respond when the Spirit moves me in that direction.

At the same rate I do play a vital role in the session. By the grace of God I am able to use wisdom and discernment to suspect when patients' pain problems are emotionally or spiritually driven. Largely I suspect emotional issues when medical tests (imaging, etc.) are negative or if the patient fails to respond to reasonable treatment. But sometimes I just get a gut feeling from the Holy Spirit that the patient needs counseling. And then my Counselor, the Holy Spirit, gives me the right words and lets it all happen.

I normally offer inner healing to only a tiny percentage of my patients (those who are willing and/or able to receive it), and maybe only once or twice during the period of months or years in which I treat them. The method is so powerful that more sessions aren't necessary in the vast majority of cases.

When I do offer inner healing, I generally do so in conjunction with traditional medical interventions, such as manual medicine, and it is only with the patient's express permission. As you have seen from other examples in this book, I pray, dialogue, and work on the patient's tissue tension at the same time. Talk about multitasking, right? This unique approach allows me to facilitate healing in the patient's mind, body, and spirit all at once—and fast too.

Clearing the Spiritual Atmosphere

At the beginning of the inner healing encounter I clear my mind and clear the spiritual atmosphere of the room through prayer. Sometimes I pray silently, and at other times I pray out loud so the patient can hear. I generally ask God to forgive both me and my patient, as we are sinners. I ask for mercy and ask God to help us forgive those we hold grudges against. And I express my faith in God and praise Him for His goodness.

My prayer might sound something like this: "Lord, You said that where two or more are gathered, You'd be in their midst. Well, [patient's name] and I are gathered in Your presence, and we believe You're going to show up. You also said we could ask for anything in line with Your will and receive it. Well, we're asking for healing knowledge so that [patient's name] can experience freedom from [name the bothersome emotion or physical problem]."

If led by the Spirit to do so, I also say words similar to what my pastor-friend Quinn Schipper advocates, "In the name of Jesus and by the blood of Jesus, I command any forces that are unhealthy, unholy, and unintended by God to be eliminated from this environment so that [my patient's name] can receive knowledge and healing."

Once the air is cleared, I then invite God, Jesus, and the Holy Spirit to be at the center of the experience so as to guide us to excellent healing for the patient in mind, body, and spirit.

Finding the Hurt Inner Child

My next step is to help the patient capture and identify the unwanted emotion that is contributing to his or her pain. I might ask, "If you had to label the emotion you feel when you experience that physical pain, what would you call it? Is it fear or anger, low self-esteem, or some other emotion?" I like to give the patient a long multiple-choice list so as to not plant ideas in his or her head.

After my patient identifies the prevailing current emotion (anxiety, for instance), I ask him to identify the earliest age at which he felt the same emotion. Sometimes the patient recalls a vivid, unpleasant memory, such as, "When I was ten, my family life fell apart." At that point I ask my adult patient to close his eyes and picture himself at this age. I have the patient make eye contact, if possible, with his younger self and try to read what he is feeling or thinking.

Usually I get answers such as these: "Daddy was drinking." "My parents got a divorce." "My brothers and sisters used to tell me I was stupid." "The kids at school were bullying me." "Uncle Jimmy touched me." And so on. Then I start talking to the inner child through my patient, as the patient maintains eye contact in his imagination.

I ask my patient's inner child if he knows who I am. If the child says (through the adult patient), "No," I introduce myself. I then ask the child if he knows Jesus, and the answer varies. If the child doesn't know Jesus, I explain who He is, and at some point in the session, I invite him to know the Lord.

Interestingly the adult patient sometimes speaks to me with the voice of a child as he or she relates what the inner child is thinking or feeling. The patient's voice changes in loudness and strength, and the patient actually sounds like a child. It's really cool when this happens. You can read more about this phenomenon in *Trading Faces*. Pastor Schipper calls these different childlike personas "alters," as in alter egos.

Identifying the Lies;
Asking God to Reveal the Truth

It's important to keep the discussion age-appropriate when talking with the patient's inner child. I speak with forty-year-olds differently than I speak with five-year-olds. But no matter the age of the child, I keep the discussion focused on God as the generator of truth and the devil as the generator of lies.

I explain how God wants us to feel peace and joy, whereas the devil (also known as the accuser) wants to harm us with lies, such as "You're fat," "You're ugly," "You're stupid," etc. (Again, I usually recite a long list of lies in random order, because I don't want to introduce false perceptions into the mind of the inner child.)

I then ask my patient's inner child if the accuser has lied to him or her in any of the ways I mentioned or in any other way. I might say something like, "Earlier, you told me your daddy drinks and hits your mom. Do you think there are any lies the devil wants you to believe about yourself because of what's going on in your life?"

The child might respond by saying, "It's my fault that Daddy is mad," or "If I weren't stupid and got bad grades, Daddy wouldn't be mad," or "I'm just a bad kid." If the patient is able to identify the lie, I encourage him or her. I say, "Those sound exactly like lies the devil would want you to believe."

Then I go on to say, "What do you think the truth is if that's the lie. What would God tell you? God always tells the truth." Then I pray and ask God to reveal the truth about this painful situation to my patient. That's when the patient typically says something like, "It's not my fault? I'm not stupid? I'm not bad?"

"Right!" I'd then say, "Now, who would God say you are? The devil said you're stupid and bad. But how would God describe you? What or who does God say you are?"

It's extremely important to help the patient's inner child realize his or her true identity in Christ. You have to know your true identity to be able to tell when the devil lies to you! That's why I ask, "Who or what does *God* say you are?"

Interestingly in most cases the truth comes in the form of a question, not a statement. You can hear it in the patient's tone of voice. "I'm a caring and capable person? I'm not stupid or bad?"

"Absolutely," I'd reply.

Sometimes the truth is not the direct opposite of the lie, either. If the lie was, "You're bad," the truth might be, "You're mine" or, "You're delightful," instead of "You're good." Recall that's what happened in my own embryo and fetus visions.

Ultimate Healing Through Forgiveness

By itself, the revelation of truth from God to the patient (plus the revelation of his or her true identity, i.e., "I am a caring and capable person") is tremendously healing. But there's still another step, and this last step is even more healing than being purged of the lies. The next step has to do with forgiveness.

In this step I explain to the child about how hurt people hurt people, and I inquire about what the child knows about his or her abuser's childhood. Most of the time the child says something like, "Daddy's father used to beat him." When the child acknowledges that the person who hurt him also was hurt as a child, it becomes easier to forgive that person.

If the patient still won't forgive the other person, I explain how forgiveness doesn't justify the abuser's actions or get him off the hook with God. No matter what, the abuser will still have to answer to God on judgment day. I try to explain that continued unforgiveness hurts only the patient.

Most of the time the patient comes around and forgives his or her abuser, but sometimes the person just can't forgive (yet). As I said before, this is directed by God, not me. I may have a loose "model" in mind for how to run a person through this "talking to the inner child," but I don't schedule God, and I can't make anyone forgive anybody to receive anything if he or she doesn't want to.

Deliverance Can Augment Inner Healing

Sometimes my patients' problems are due to other factors besides misperceptions and lies they believe about themselves due to traumatic past experiences. Sometimes people have "bad juju" on them, spiritually. OK, I admit I borrowed that word *juju* from one of my doctor friends. I think you know what I mean, though. Some people have spiritual garbage on them due to their sins, their ancestors' sins, or other things that are almost too creepy to think about, and those spiritual forces lead to bad things happening in their lives. Those people often benefit from what is called "deliverance."

To help you understand what I mean by deliverance, allow me to give you a paraphrased definition. In a nutshell deliverance is when you prayerfully cast out of demons in Jesus's name. I believe that once you accept Jesus as your Savior, you can't actually be "possessed" by demons and be made to spew up green pea soup like young Linda Blair in *The Exorcist*. However, you can still be highly irritated and annoyed by oppressive spiritual forces that descend on you at times.

The Bible is full of examples of how demons can oppress people and make them sick. If you don't believe bad spirits exist and complicate lives, just go to the BibleGateway.com, where the Bible is available online in a multitude of translations, and search the word *demon*. You'll find dozens of scriptures that talk about how Jesus cast out demons from sick and emotionally tortured people.

Deliverance vs. Inner Healing

A pastor-friend explained the difference between deliverance and Christian inner healing to me this way: "Without the lies, the demons can't latch onto you. Get rid of the lies, and the demons that attach to those lies will leave you alone." In other words, deliverance may work for a while, but if you don't address the underlying lies that those demons are attracted to (via inner healing, prayer, or some other method), you're likely to keep attracting new demons.

My pastor-friend, who hails from a Methodist background, used this example: "If you leave a bowl of honey on the table, flies will swarm around it." In his analogy the honey is like the lies you believe about yourself, and the flies are like the demons that are attracted to those lies.

My friend went on to say, "If you spend your energy and attention on chasing those flies away [as we cast off demons in Jesus's name via deliverance], your solution may be only temporary, because even if you kill the ones that are currently attracted to the honey, new ones will come once those are gone. Just get rid of the honey. Then the flies will become uninterested and they'll leave, looking for honey elsewhere."

I believe that inner healing works even better than deliverance for some people, though the approaches can overlap and both can be helpful. Thus, don't be surprised if your highly experienced counselor, pastor, or therapist uses a combination of deliverance and inner healing (and maybe even a few other techniques) during your session. For more information about deliverance, as well as leads for finding a deliverance minister in your area, contact the International Society of Deliverance Ministers.

Directories of Christian Counselors

Though I personally counsel a small minority of my patients, I believe many of them would benefit from more intense counseling than what I can provide in a twenty-minute doctor's appointment. So I refer patients to ministers and counselors quite frequently. Sometimes I send patients to Christian counselors who have master's and doctoral degrees, and other times I send patients to lay ministers. It really just depends on how the Spirit moves me in the case of each individual patient.

Below you will find the names of three directories of Christian counselors that I have accessed in the past. You may also find counselors by looking in your local phone book or by performing an Internet search for Christian counselors in your geographic area. Feel free to call potential counselors, and if you believe inner healing is right for you, ask them if they employ inner healing as one of their counseling tools. However, don't dismiss a counselor just because he or she does not offer inner healing. God works through a variety of counseling languages, depending on the skill level and gift set of the individual counselor (and the needs of the client).

For example, I have heard many positive responses from patients who have undergone what is called "EMDR" (a therapy that involves certain orchestrated eye movements) for dealing with past emotional trauma. Some of my patients have even undergone a combination of inner healing and EMDR with excellent results. As I said, don't put God in a box, because He may heal you in a variety of ways that you don't expect.

American Association of Christian Counselors
P. O. Box 739
Forest, VA 24551
800-526-8673
434-525-9470
www.aacc.net

National Christian Counselors Association
5260 Paylor Lane
Sarasota, FL 34240
941-388-6868
www.ncca.org

Christian Counselors Directory
3931 Mary-Eliza Trace NW
Suite 210, PMB 160
Marietta, GA 30064
800-218-8189
www.ChristianTherapist.com

What About Secular Counseling?

Since you're reading this book, I assume that your Christian faith is a big part of your life and you rely on it to help you through life's difficult times. Thus I am going to assume you would prefer a Christian counselor over a secular one. There's no substitute for having that common ground of spiritual understanding.

But what if you live where you can't find a formally trained Christian counselor? Or what if no Christian counselors are covered on your health insurance plan? Many of my patients fall into this category, depending on where they live and what kind of insurance benefits they hold.

Rest assured that God can use secular counselors to heal you. God can heal you using anybody He chooses, no matter what health insurance plan you subscribe to, and no matter who your preferred providers are. If God can speak to man through a donkey, He can use secular counselors to heal you. (I don't mean that in a judgmental way; I mean only that God is not limited in the same way that people are limited.) Just find fellow Christians to pray with you for your healing and that your counselor will be led by the Spirit to give you good advice.

Chapter 21

LET GOD SPEAK INTO
YOUR IMAGINATION

As Andy neared the end of his medical treatment, he still had unexplained neck pain. The MRI was negative, the trigger point injections weren't working, and we ruled out his rotator cuff as the cause. I even did OMM on him a few times with no success. So I asked him about emotional stress that might be contributing to his pain.

Like most patients, Andy first admitted the "less personal" layers of stress, such as work and money. But eventually he told me about the biggest stressor of his life. When Andy was only five years old, he lost his father in a freak car accident. I don't remember the details, but I understood that some car part malfunctioned and led to the crash.

Because Andy's body tensed up when he told me about this, I could tell it was adding physical strain to his body. So I pursued the issue by dialoguing with him about it. You can't throw me a bone like that and expect me to ignore it.

While I worked on Andy's neck problem, I asked him to close his eyes and try to make eye contact with the image of his five-year-old self. I thought we could try again to talk with Little Andy to help Big Andy release some emotional and physical tension.

Unfortunately Andy wasn't able to make eye contact with his younger self in his imagination. I could see he was getting frustrated. So I finally said, "It's OK. We don't have to try talking to your inner child anymore. Let me just stick to the straight physical OMM work on your neck one last time. If it doesn't work, I'll just have to release you because I've done everything I can do and can't fix you. I'm sorry."

At that point the weirdest thing happened. As soon as I closed my eyes so I could better concentrate on what I felt on Andy's neck, God painted an image of five-year-old Andy in *my* mind. What happened after that was truly amazing.

In this chapter I tell you the rest of Andy's story. I also encourage you to open your imagination to God. Let Him speak to you in unexpected ways. He may paint visual images, or He may give you audible words, thoughts, physical sensations, or even emotions that contribute to your understanding and emotional healing. It really just depends on the way in which He knows you best receive.

In the vision (which occurred purely in my imagination) little five-year-old Andy desperately flung his arms around my neck like he was trying to keep from drowning. I saw the urgency in his face and *felt* (not heard) him broadcast, "Don't leave me!"

Little Andy buried his little face in my neck and held on to me for dear life. That's when he began to cry. It was a wailing, groaning, exhausted, suffering cry that emanated from the depths of his soul.

Though it seemed to last forever, Little Andy's emotional catharsis probably lasted only five minutes of "earth" time. At the end of it, I still had my hands on grown-up Andy's neck since I was still doing OMM on him.

Let me reiterate something before I go on. The "talking to the inner child" thing is not actually a normal part of OMM. It's just something I like to do it because it magnifies the patients' relief. It addresses the patients' emotional and spiritual issues at the same time as the OMM techniques address their physical issues. It's like triple-teaming the problem. Now, getting back to Andy...

About the time I felt the abnormal tension in Andy's neck start to decrease, little five-year-old Andy stopped crying in my imagination. Coincidentally that was the same moment my patient said his neck was beginning to feel better.

As if it couldn't get cooler, Grownup Andy's neck suddenly popped back into place and thereafter the tension in his neck completely normalized. I had been trying to get it to do that (indirectly) for three visits, but it wouldn't pop until after Andy let go of that pent-up emotion that was keeping his neck tense and out of alignment.

Meanwhile, God and I Were Talking...

During the five minutes that Little Andy balled his eyes out in my imagination, I had a little side conversation with God. "Did you do this, Lord? Or did I imagine it without You? I wonder if the 'other' guy put it in my mind to throw me off. Maybe I'm just going off the deep end."

I didn't really need to ask Him for confirmation. I already knew the truth. I wasn't capable of conceiving such an amazing vision on my own. It was as mind-blowing as the "Fetus Rita" vision. Unexpected healing miracles like that come only from God. As it says in 1 Corinthians 2:9 "No eye has seen, no ear has heard, no mind has conceived what God has prepared for those who love him."

Because I knew the vision was from God, I reluctantly went on to ask, "Do I have to tell him, Lord?" The answer was, "Yes," but that's not the answer I wanted. I already told Andy we didn't have to talk with his inner child again, and I didn't want to go back on my word. I wanted to hear God say, "No, don't tell him," so I asked again. "Do I have to tell him, Lord?" Unfortunately the answer was still yes. "But Lord, I don't even know if he even believes..."

I'm sure you can understand why I was reluctant. It was a frankly weird experience. Plus I have a reputation to uphold with my fellow physicians, and I didn't know what other doctors he might tell. But God confirmed that I was to tell him, so I did.

Thankfully I no longer care what people think of me. That's why I'm now telling the whole world about the awesome and unexpected ways in which God heals people.

Why Andy Couldn't Receive Without Help

God communicated with me in a completely new way in this situation with Andy. He created the healing in my mind and worked through me because apparently Little Andy was not able to receive the healing by his own accord. You may have heard it said, "God meets you where you are." In this case God met *me* where Andy was so I could help him get out of that place.

I later found out why Andy had all that pent-up grief in him over his father's death. He never fully grieved over his loss. Andy was the youngest of six children. Unfortunately his widowed, grieving mother couldn't attend to his emotional needs, as she too was grieving and she had five other kids to care for yet no money or energy to do it. Believe it or not, the first time Andy cried over losing his dad was the day he cried in *my* imagination.

I guess the five-year-old part of him who retained this trauma was too young and too wounded to actively participate. Or maybe I just didn't have the right words to initiate an actual verbal conversation with Little Andy. On second thought, maybe there were no right words.

Tools and Weapons

I have been blessed to observe or participate in inner healing sessions offered by various types of practitioners, including Christian psychologists with PhDs and ordained and lay Christian ministers. Interestingly no matter which type of practitioner guided the experience, I noticed a common denominator. God tended to work through visual images. He gave the participants images of tools and weapons in their imaginations for use in combating the accuser's lies.

In one experience, with his eyes closed and in a state of expectant prayer, the person being counseled received an image of a wall that separated him from God. On recognition of the wall the minister led the counselee in a prayer, asking God to give him a tool to break down the wall. Within ten seconds the man blurted out, "It's a jackhammer!" As soon as the jackhammer broke through the wall, the man could see sunlight on the other side.

Later in the same session (since residual barriers were still present), the minister asked God to give the man another tool to more fully tear down the wall. The second time around the tool was a bulldozer. It completely demolished the rest of the wall and pushed away the rubble as well, so the man could finally see the truth on the other side of the wall.

In still other experiences that I observed, a person plagued with fear was given a mighty silver dagger to beat down his worries and anxieties. And still another person was given a shield to cover the part of his body in which he carried his stress (his back). God communicates with us in countless different ways.

Shedding Unneeded Garments

You probably know that it's common for people to have body image issues even after they lose weight. They continue to feel like ponderous elephants, even if they look entirely "normal" (whatever "normal" means). That was sure true in my case. For many years after I lost weight I continued to feel too fat. Finally it dawned on me that I could ask God for help so I could see myself the way He sees me and feel more peace in my mind and less physical tension in my body.

Because of my prayer God "fixed" something in the spiritual realm that I don't understand. I'm not sure, but I think He removed something that was appended to me. I suspect it was a lie that I believed about myself or an irrational fear I'd carried around since childhood. Either way, the result was that I no longer needed to perceive myself as overweight.

I knew I was different after that prayer because after God fixed me, I looked down (in my mind's eye) and saw that my skin had come loose, as though I was wearing a giant overall garment that was flesh-colored and made of squishy fat. That's when I had the urge to reach down to my ankles and pull the garment up over my head like I was skinning a rabbit. I threw the garment of fat away and found my underlying smaller body that matched my real body size.

No-Strings-Attached Forgiveness

My pastor-friend Quinn Schipper, the author of the Christian inner healing books *Trading Faces* and *The Language of Forgiveness*, gave me permission to use one of his visual aids for your benefit.

In the first of the two sessions I had with Quinn, he talked with my inner child about an event that occurred when I was seven years old. Quinn helped me get to the point of extending forgiveness to a person whom I perceived to have hurt me. But when I reached the crossroads where I could either forgive or hang onto the bitterness, I didn't want to forgive the person at first.

Quinn said, "If it helps, you can imagine a little red string that binds you to the person. In your mind's eye, take a pair of scissors and cut the string while saying, [so-and-so], I forgive you."

Quinn wanted me to release the person with no expectation of an apology or that the other person would even be able to realize or comprehend how I felt or what he or she did wrong. It was "no strings attached" forgiveness. I was to cut the string and release the person to God, allowing Him to deal with punishment (or forgiveness) as He saw fit.

Quinn actually had me say, "I forgive you," out loud as I cut the string in my imagination. After I did so, the person just floated away in my imagination, and I felt the Holy Spirit just wash over me and release me from the weight of unforgiveness.

When I counsel my own patients toward forgiveness, I use a modified version of Quinn's string analogy. I tell them to imagine several strings, some in one color (such as red) and the others in a different color (such as orange). I have the patient assign one color to the "bad" strings and another color to the "good" strings. (I chose red and orange because my office is in Norman, Oklahoma. Anybody who knows Big Twelve college sports knows what the colors red and orange stand for in my neck of the woods.)

After my patients see the people they wish to forgive in their imaginations and the strings that attach them together, I ask the patients to cut whichever color of strings they want to cut. Some patients want to cut all the strings because they want nothing to do with the people who hurt them, and others choose to cut only one of the two colors. That way they can retain the good parts of the person who hurt them and let the rest float away.

Right after that the images of the people to be forgiven generally disappear from the patients' minds and they feel calmer and happier. Additionally, by whichever colors they choose to cut, I can figure out which team they root for. In turn, that helps me decide if I really want to help them or if I just want to give them placebos.

How to Be in Chaos But Not Part of It

When Julie, a doctoral student, visits her dysfunctional family, she uses specific mental techniques to detach emotionally so she doesn't get entangled in family conflict and strife. I didn't make this up—she did—and she gave me permission to write about her idea.

As Julie interacts with her family in conversation, she gets into a mental state that sounds to me like an out-of-body experience. She becomes like an impartial observer—more like the narrator of the family story rather than an actual character in the story.

By all outward appearances Julie appears to interact with her family in the usual way during these get-togethers. She makes eye contact, engages with them, and smiles as she talks. But internally she said she detaches. Meanwhile she tells herself things that help her cope. She reminds herself that "hurt people hurt people," and that it's biblical to turn the other cheek when her family members say inflammatory things.

Her internal dialogue sounds like this: "You [referring to the person she is talking to] don't realize you're anxious, do you?" "You insulted me only because you feel threatened." Or, "You chose chaos and strife but I choose God and peace," and, "I wish I could help you, but you still aren't able to receive."

Let me repeat that she doesn't actually say these things out loud. She merely thinks them in her mind, and she does so with an attitude of love and compassion. She also prays, "Thank You, Jesus, for helping me to feel peace. Someday please let me help my family find what I found in You. Until then please continue to help me let their comments go in one ear and out the other."

Perhaps you could pray about finding your own technique for

dealing with people who stir up your negative emotions in those times when you can't avoid those people. The trick is to be creative and use your imagination to find ways to be *in* the chaotic world without being *of* the chaotic world.

Trash Cans in Your Mind

One of my pain-management patients uses an interesting technique for stress management. In his imagination he visualizes putting his troubles into a trash can, and then he imagines leaving the trash can at the curb for the garbage trucks to pick up.

He graciously offered his imagery tool for your benefit. But if you prefer, tweak it to make it your own. For example, you can imagine leaving your container of worries at the altar, where you can present it to God as an act of trust and worship, saying, "Lord, I choose to release my strife to You and trade it for peace."

Or imagine your worries to be rocks that you carry in a backpack. In your mind's eye imagine that you are in the Lord's presence, and offer each rock to Him out of your backpack as an act of submission. "Dear Jesus, now I release the burden of unforgiveness toward my first husband." Then visualize Jesus removing that stone from your backpack and feel how much lighter the pack becomes!

God communicates with you in any way you can receive it because He is merciful. Just open your imagination to Him, and see how He responds!

Chapter 22

CHOOSE TRUTH OVER LIES

IMAGINE WE'RE ALIKE in more ways than you think. I don't like physical pain, and I don't like feeling hungry or thirsty for too long. That's why I can't even imagine how awful it must have been for Jesus to go without food for forty days. Seriously! Think about that. *Forty days without food.*

By the time the devil tempted Him at the end of the fast, any other human would have been at the minimum mentally delirious, if not dead. But Jesus had the presence of mind to rise above His physical weakness and respond with God's Word.

> After fasting forty days and forty nights, he was hungry. The tempter came to him and said, "If you are the Son of God, tell these stones to become bread." Jesus answered, "It is written: 'Man does not live on bread alone, but on every word that comes from the mouth of God.'"
>
> —MATTHEW 4:2-4

Each of the three times the devil lied, Jesus refuted the lies with specific truth from the Old Testament. Did you hear what I said? Even in His most vulnerable state, Jesus used Scripture as truth and power against the devil's accusations. He didn't combat the devil's lies on His own strength.

Just as Jesus did, you must capture the lies when they are hurled at you in your everyday life and refute them with truth as it appears in Scripture. No matter what your resultant emotions tell you and no matter how weak and vulnerable you feel, discipline yourself to grab the lies by the throat and hold them up against the wall of truth.

Let the lie's arms and legs struggle in futile helplessness as you hold it up off the ground by the throat. Then watch the lie weaken and finally wither away and vanish, just as the devil vanished when Jesus spoke God's Word in his presence. There you go. Feel free to use that visual aid the next time you feel attacked by the enemy. Hold the enemy up against the wall of truth using Scripture.

In this chapter I give you a framework for how to use Scripture as a tool so you can better grab your personal lies by the throat and lift them up to Scripture for correction. You didn't know I had that much testosterone in me, did you? Grrrrr!!!

The Importance of Identifying Your Emotions

In the self-talk exercise I describe in this chapter, I give you a core statement to say out loud: "I choose to ignore my [pick a word to describe your unwanted emotion: depression, anxiety, anger, etc.] and instead focus on God's truth in this situation."

Having to fill in the blank requires you to identify and name your emotion. What emotion do you feel at the moment you're tempted to reach for your false comforter? Is it anger, frustration, weakness, shame, helplessness, or hopelessness? Do you feel anxious or out of control? Some emotion likely triggers you. I force you to name it.

It sounds like a small point, but it's actually a very big one. Many people are oblivious to their emotions. Instead of acknowledging and feeling them, they habitually escape them by reaching for distractions in the form of false comforters. Or they transform their emotions into pain or physical illness because, in some way, it feels less threatening to think, "My back hurts" or, "I can't stand this irritable bowel syndrome," rather than, "I feel vulnerable."

If you've been an emotional eater for your whole life, or if you're used to medicating your emotions with false comforters, then forcing yourself to name your unwanted emotions can be therapeutic in itself. When you name your emotions, you can deal with them much more easily.

Give your emotion a name so it becomes tangible. It's hard to battle an enemy that doesn't have a face. When you give your emotion a name, you give a face to the enemy (and even a body). Then you can, as I said earlier, pick it up by the throat and hold it against the truth of God's truth for comparison.

The Healing Touch

Sometimes negative emotions are stored in body parts. Some people feel stress in their backs and necks, in the form of headaches, stomachaches, unexplained rashes, hot flashes, and even bowel and bladder problems.

If you're one of those people whose stress becomes actual physical pain or illness, you may benefit from holding, rubbing, or tapping on your physical sore spot as you recite the positive affirmations in this chapter. I asked a psychologist colleague why she thinks this works for some people. She said she thinks it helps divide a person's attention so he or she can approach an uncomfortable memory or emotion more closely.

In other words, without the physical distraction some people find it too difficult to deal with their emotional pain. I guess it's like distracting a patient with a funny story while I jab them with a needle to give them a shot.

In pain management we utilize a tool called "counter stimulation" to lessen the perception of pain. It involves using an electrical device called a TENS unit. TENS is an acronym for "transcutaneous electrical nerve stimulation." You attach the unit to your painful area with electrodes and then the unit sends a tingly sensation into your skin. That tingle sensation is carried to your spinal cord, and it blocks the pain signals from traveling up the spinal cord to the brain. It's a way to lessen your physical pain by generating an electrical distraction.

Counter-stimulation is like when a dog hurts his paw and then licks it. Or like when you rub a body part that you just injured. The nonpainful stimulus competes with the painful stimulus in getting the attention of your brain. You have a hard time focusing on your first pain when you feel the second sensation as well.

Am I suggesting that you lick your foot while you pray so you can better deal with your childhood trauma? No. The reason is you probably can't reach your foot because you're too overweight and out of shape, and I don't want you to strain your back when you bend over, because then I'd have to fix you.

Fortunately for some people merely holding, rubbing, or tapping on an emotionally charged body part (or a neutral body part) during the self-talk exercise can accomplish the same type of counter-stimulation. The touch stimulus divides your attention from your painful emotions, just as my psychologist colleague hypothesized. That way you can approach your painful emotion more closely because you're semi-distracted.

If you don't feel comfortable touching or rubbing a painful body part as you read though this, just skip it! Engage in just the positive self-talk part if you want. It's completely your choice.

Getting Into Your Body

Do you live in your mind more than your heart or your actual physical body? Sometimes this happens in cases of significant past trauma. Maybe you feel emotionally "shell-shocked" due to things that happened to you in the past, and that leads you to feel emotionally disconnected, as if you're just going through the motions of life alone.

In a way, retreating into your mind is like a defense mechanism. Your mind stops receiving messages from your body and emotions because those areas make you feel vulnerable. I heard that's true for a lot of the Holocaust survivors. They were emotionally numb and unable to "connect" with other people after their trauma. They just went through the motions of life without feeling strong emotion—at least that's what their kids frequently complained of.

If this is the case for you, then holding an emotionally charged body part during your prayer time might help you. It can help you to wake up your body and function as a more integrated being.

What defines an "emotionally charged" body part? If you had to get stitches on your forehead as a child and the emergency room visit scared you, or if your ex-abuser used to punch your head, your head might be an emotionally charged area. In that case you might decide to hold your forehead as you call on those old, painful memories. The physical touch could be very healing to your inner, hurt child.

Another example of an emotionally charged body part might be your neck or back if those areas tense up when you're under stress. There is no right or wrong answer regarding what body part carries meaning for you, as it depends entirely on your experience, which is unique.

At this point, since we're almost ready to get started, let me mention a disclaimer about the self-talk exercise that follows. Pray strongly about whether or not the sample exercise in this chapter is right for you, and proceed *only* if you're in the presence of a licensed counselor or pastor who can guide you. If you proceed without professional guidance, you do so at your own risk!

Before You Start the Exercise

To prepare yourself, before you start the exercise:

- **Have an attitude of submission before God.** You are not the healer here, and you bear no responsibility for guiding the healing process. You are merely presenting yourself to God for Him to guide you.

- **Show your faith.** State your affirmations with a tone of voice that reflects that you mean business. You believe that God is healing you, right? Then your tone should reflect that. Get excited! Be strong! Make your statements boldly. Stomp on the accuser's lies.

- **Remember this is all about prayer.** This is not a standardized test that you pass or fail, and it's not a cookbook recipe for "freedom from bondage." However, if you don't know where to start on your own, you may wish to include some or all of these components in your prayer.

- Invite Jesus to be in the center of your healing.

- Apologize for your sins.

- God said you could ask for anything in line with His will and He would give it to you. So ask for healing knowledge, wisdom, and mercy!

- Express your thankfulness.

- Clear the spiritual atmosphere. In the name of Jesus command all unholy forces—anything unintended by God to be there (fear, anxiety, anger, depression, addiction, perfectionism, generational bondage, etc.)—to be bound and eliminated from the environment.

- Ask God to reveal barriers or lies, false burdens, confusion, etc., that have influenced your thinking.

- Ask God to reveal His healing truth that refutes those lies.

- Ask for help to extend forgiveness to those who hurt you. It's critical for your healing.

The Self-Talk Scripture Exercise

1. *Rate the intensity of your negative emotions* (such as fear, anger, nervousness, compulsion to reach for your favorite false comforter, etc.) at the outset of the exercise. On a scale of zero to ten one is very little negative emotion and ten is maximally intense negative emotion. You will rerate the intensity later.

2. *Assess whether you feel physical pain.* If you are experiencing pain, you may or may not decide to touch that

part. Perhaps God's healing will flow through your hand during the exercise. Try to relax the body part so it releases tension.

3. *Say your core statement out loud:* "I choose to ignore this false emotion so I can focus on truth." Say it with emphasis, like you mean it (no matter how you actually feel), repeating it five to seven times for reinforcement.

4. *Now take a huge, deep, cleansing breath all the way in and all the way out.* Exhale your stress and tension and negative emotion, and thank God for His goodness. Let your shoulders down and relax as though you are a rag doll. Now rerate the intensity of your negative emotion on a scale of zero to ten. Did it go down?

5. *Repeat the godly affirmations, adding Scripture* (see Appendix B for relevant verses). Say, "I choose to ignore this false emotion so I can focus on truth. The Lord delivers me from my problems" (Ps. 34:4), or "By His wounds I am healed" (Isa. 53:5). Say this repeatedly and with emphasis. After you speak, breathe in God's truth and breathe out the lies. Rerate your negative emotions on a scale of one to ten. Has your emotion become less severe?

6. *If you still feel the bothersome emotion or urge, repeat the affirmation, again with Scripture.* For example, "I choose to ignore this false emotion so I can focus on truth. Lord, You said I could ask for and receive anything in prayer. So I ask for and receive freedom from this unwanted emotion. Thank You, Jesus." As before, take a big breath in and out, exhale your unwanted emotion, and relax your shoulders. Rerate your emotion. Is it more than zero? If so, continue.

7. *If you still feel the unwanted emotion,* consider adding to your statement, "I choose to ignore this false emotion

so I can focus on truth. I don't really crave [name your false comforter]. I crave 'pure spiritual milk' (1 Pet. 2:2). Thank You, Lord, for giving me real satisfaction." Repeat several times. Take a big cleansing breath. Rerate your level of emotional discomfort.

8. *Now add even more truth, if you wish.* Say, "I choose to ignore this false emotion so I can focus on truth. Through the blood of Jesus I am a new creation, and I receive God's forgiveness and peace." Repeat several times. Breathe in God's forgiveness and breathe out guilt and shame. There is no condemnation in Christ.

9. *After the emotion or urge reaches or gets very close to the zero point (total release), move on to forgiveness*: "I choose to ignore this false emotion so I can focus on truth. Just as I have received God's mercy, I now choose to extend it. Lord, I release [insert a name here] to You, with no expectation of apology or payback." Then give a big inhalation and exhalation, relax your shoulders, and open and lift your hands (if you want) to demonstrate that you are giving your emotional burden to the Lord.

10. *Repeat the affirmation statement one last time*, saying, "I choose to ignore this false emotion so I can focus on truth. Now I choose to let go of this emotion and give it to the Lord. Thank You, Jesus, for taking it away from me." Inhale and exhale deeply, relax your neck and shoulders, lift your *open* hands up to the Lord, envision Him taking your burden, and thank Him as that burden floats away from you. Finally consider journaling, singing praise to God, or resting in a spirit of thanksgiving.

Additional Notes About
How to Use the Above Exercise

Notice how your affirmation is action-oriented. You're *choosing* to side with God and *focusing* on truth rather than the accuser's lies. "I choose to ignore the false emotion so I can focus on truth." This is all about your choosing to believe what is right and true and acting on it rather than believing the lies that manipulated your emotions in the past.

Scripture is the most important part: "I choose to ignore the false emotion and focus on truth. Therefore I choose to believe [then quote Scripture]." Remember, you're not fighting the emotion on your own strength. You're fighting with truth.

And don't say, "*my*" false emotion, because if you keep saying it's yours, you might decide to keep it! Say, "*the*" false emotion, instead. Always remember to take the big cleansing breath after your statements, let go of your physical tension (drop and relax your shoulders too), and thank and praise God for the help.

Chapter 23

YOUR TRUE IDENTITY

A s you might guess, I'm a talker, and that comes in handy if I'm giving you painful injections. I can distract even the most anxious patient with my lawyer jokes and other entertaining stories. "Do you know why sharks don't eat lawyers? Professional courtesy." That's one of my all-time favorites. And believe it or not, I got it from a patient who happens to be an attorney.

Patients think it's humane of me to distract them during injections, but the truth is it's for my benefit too. Not only am I female, but also I'm an *Italian* female. I'm genetically programmed to talk. If you bound my mouth with masking tape, I'd be forced to talk with my hands, and that's the last thing you want me to do when I'm wielding a spinal needle in a sterile surgical field.

On a good day, in the midst of the inane but amusing verbiage, I somehow manage to spew out words of spiritual wisdom. If God can talk through a donkey, as He did in the Bible, He can certainly talk through me when I'm in the spiritual groove with Him. My favorite example happened a couple years ago when I saw a back pain patient who I could tell felt lowly, stupid, ugly, and worthless. I literally felt her depression through the words she spoke as well as by her physical posture.

As I worked on this patient, I felt overcome with a thought from God. Without thinking too much about it (which is how I come up with my best material), I blurted out, "You have to know who you are to know who you *aren't*."

It's hard to deflect lies when you don't even recognize them as lies. You must know who you are in Christ if you want to be able to deflect the false accusations (and/or reject negative thoughts that spring from your own mind). Let me repeat this because it's important. When you know who you are, you also know who you aren't.

The French mathematician and philosopher Blaise Pascal said it like this: "Not only do we not know God except through Jesus Christ; we do not even know ourselves except through Jesus Christ."[1]

It's only through Christ's loving and forgiving eyes that we can see ourselves as we really are. We're too biased and flawed (not to mention unforgiving) to make accurate assessments of ourselves. We can't know who we are without God's grace showing us who we are. In this chapter please let me remind you who God says you are. That way you can better reject the lies that lead to physical illness, stress, unwanted behaviors, and physical pain.

Your New Name Is "Beloved"

If you haven't already done so, it's time to reject the old names you once answered to. Thankfully, even if you committed sin, God never saw you as *being* your sin. If anything the opposite is true. God hates the sin but loves the sinner.

I'm not a Bible expert, but it seems that God saves the derogatory labels for self-righteous hypocrites such as the Pharisees (Jewish religious leaders), whom He called "a brood of snakes" (Matt. 23:33, NLT). They had planks sticking out of their own eyes (representing major hypocrisy and sin) while trying to pick specks out of others' eyes.

As good and merciful as God is, know that He prefers to send you down the path of emotional healing and forgiveness without labeling you or in any way equating you with your sin. If He does give you a name, it'll be something good and positive, such as "Beloved" or, as it was in my case, "Delightful."

"I [God] Will Tell You Who You Are"

Years ago tiny little voices of self-doubt tried to sabotage the healing ministry God preordained for me. The voices said, "You're a doctor, not an author; you have no business writing books." "You're a medical doctor not an osteopath; you don't belong at manipulation courses with physical therapists and doctors of osteopathy." "You're not a pastor; you have no business counseling patients spiritually." And, "You're not a specialist in psychiatry; you have no business talking about human behavior."

If I believed those statements, I wouldn't have helped nearly as many people as I have find freedom from pain, stress, obesity, or hell. Logically I knew I was more than qualified to do all the things I mentioned. I am a medical doctor, so I'm licensed to touch, treat, and counsel patients in a multitude of ways. But it wasn't logic that stood in my way. It was false emotions and lies I believed about my identity in Christ.

Believing the lies (despite my credentials), I "corrected" God: "But, God—I'm a doctor, not a [fill in the blank with however you tend to limit yourself]." I felt like Dr. McCoy from *Star Trek*, "I'm a doctor, not a magician!"[2]

Thankfully God set me straight. He said, "Don't tell Me what you are. I'll tell you what you are. I can make you anything I want to you to be, and I made you a healer."

God also told me, "Use every tool I gave you," meaning, use the medicines, the MRIs, the X-rays, the shots, the talking, the writing, the OMM, the nerve tests, and the praying with patients. Different people need different things, and healers do best when they have wisdom about who needs regular medical treatment and who needs deliverance or other counseling.

That's when I received the epiphany. If God can use little children, hairdressers, and bank tellers as spiritual healers, and if He can talk through donkeys, why can't He anoint a board-certified medical subspecialist like me with special, supernatural healing gifts that transcend my medical training? The subsequent eight hundred-plus hours of manipulation training helped as well. It's not like I expected God to magically teach me osteopathic manipulation or the art of attuning to patients emotionally. He just gave me the ability and the opportunities, and I had to do the work from there.

Don't Confuse Your Identity With Your Spiritual Gifts and Talents

Spiritual gifts and talents are great things to have, but they don't necessarily define who you are. They don't make you a "good enough" person in God's eyes, and they don't justify your existence. For example, I am not a child of God because He called me to be a healer. I am a child of God because of God's loving, forgiving nature.

Before I continue with the point I want to make in this subsection, let me digress for a minute to go over some definitions. I want to explain the difference between spiritual gifts and talents in case these concepts are new to you. Spiritual gifts are special blessings that God gives to certain people through the power of the Holy Spirit. Spiritual gifts are supposed to be shared with the church and others so that all of God's creation can benefit. They are spiritual in nature, and they are created by God, not by man.

There are at least three parts of the New Testament in which the gifts are discussed. First Corinthians 12:8–11 discusses words of wisdom (prophecy), the ability to communicate practical truth (knowledge), the ability to have faith in God, the working of miracles, prophecy, discerning of spirits, speaking in unknown foreign tongues, and the interpretation of tongues. Romans 12:3–8 discusses prophecy, healing, servanthood, teaching, exhortation, and leadership. And Ephesians 4:10–12 says that God called apostles, prophets, evangelists, pastors, and teachers to equip the church for ministry.

In case you don't know what your spiritual gifts are but would like to know, allow me to refer you to a resource that is offered by my church, Lifechurch.tv. It's called "Chazown." Pastor Craig Groeschel wrote a book by that title,[3] and there is even an online course at www.Chazown.com with a test to help you find your spiritual gifts.

I took the test and found that my gifts include knowledge, teaching, exhortation, prophecy, and leadership. There weren't any questions on there about healing, but as an aside, I know I'm a "healer" too. Chazown also showed me that my core values include authenticity, boldness, courage, creativity, grace, and humor.

Now let me shift gears and talk about talents. In contrast to spiritual gifts, which are God-given, talents are special abilities that people acquire through practice, experience, their own effort, or their genetic bloodlines. Examples of talents are the abilities to sing, play instruments, cook, draw, build things, or do the accounting for the church. Talents are important and helpful to the church, but they are not "spiritual" in nature.

Now that we're all on the same page about the meaning of "spiritual gifts" and "talents," let me tell you why it's important to know the difference. What you do for God (the offering of your gifts and talents into His service) and who you are in Christ (your identity as a Christian) are two separate things. When I say, "You have to know who you are to know who you're not," I don't necessarily mean you have to know what your gifts are or that you should base your worth and identity on your gifts and talents. I mean you need to know who God says you are.

Some people feel as if they don't know who they are in Christ. They figure if only they could discover their gifts and talents, they would finally know who they are and feel peace, security, and *value*. But that's not entirely true. They're confusing the "knowing" with the "feeling." What they really need is to feel God's love and acceptance on a deep emotional level.

To illustrate my point, let me remind you of the emotionally healing vision I had when God and I were both looking at the fetus version of me still in the womb. God kept saying, "Look at her!" as He delighted in me. However, I had no obvious gifts or talents and no ability to do anything "useful" because I was a fetus. At first I didn't understand why God adored me so much because I apparently had trouble seeing myself through His love and grace. I had a very works-oriented, hard-lined, overly pragmatic view. I saw my fetus self as being equal only to her ability to "get things done."

Boy, was I wrong. God didn't delight in me at that moment because of my future works, gifts, and talents. He delighted in me because I was His delightful creation. That was my identity at that time—simply to be His—and that was good enough for Him. Shouldn't it be good enough for you and me too?

I wish we could all accept what the Bible says in Galatians 2:16, "Know that a man is not justified by observing the law, but by faith in Jesus Christ. So we, too, have put our faith in Christ Jesus that we may be justified by faith in Christ and not by observing the law, because by observing the law no one will be justified." I love what Romans 5:1 says as well, "Therefore, since we have been justified through faith, we have peace with God through our Lord Jesus Christ."

In reality most people don't have the peace God wants them to have because they haven't yet accepted God's love all the way into their innermost places—into their identities. On one end of the spectrum are people who are tempted to define their worth by their works, and on the other end are people who feel bad about themselves for not having talents and gifts. Neither one has peace because neither has fully accepted his or her identity as already being adequate in God's eyes.

Do you see how the devil finds ways to twist even biblical concepts around to make you feel bad? He uses anything at his disposal to make you feel inadequate, even things such as spiritual gifts, which God intended to be helpful. Let me leave you a quote from an anonymous author that illustrates my point even further: "You aren't loved because you're valuable. You're valuable because God loves you."

Don't base your identity or worth on the absence or presence of your spiritual gifts and talents, your works, or any worldly measure of your value. Base your identity and worth on the fact that God loves you simply because you're His delightful creation.

What God Says About You

Read the following statements out loud. They are based on the Scripture references shown in parentheses. As you read, notice how God does not base your identity on what you have earned or on what you deserve. He bases your identity on how you look through His eyes of grace, love, and mercy. They read, "I am..." and "I have..." rather than "I do..." So boldly declare them *out loud*!

- I am fearfully and wonderfully made (Ps. 139:14).
- I have a clean conscience (Heb. 9:14; 10:17; Matt. 26:28; John 1:29).
- I am forgiven (Col. 1:14).
- I am free from condemnation (Rom. 8:1).
- I am justified by faith (Rom. 5:1).
- I am the temple of the Holy Spirit (1 Cor. 3:16).
- I am precious to God (Isa. 43:4).
- I am a new creation in Christ (2 Cor. 5:17; Eph. 4:24).
- I have been cared for since my conception (Isa. 46:3).
- I am a child of God (Rom. 8:14–15; Gal. 3:26; John 1:12).
- I am God's workmanship (Eph. 2:10).
- I am saved by grace (Eph. 2:8).
- I am born again through the Spirit of Christ (John 3:3–6).
- I am a child of light (1 Thess. 5:5).
- I am more than a conqueror through Christ (Rom. 8:37).
- I am filled with the divine nature of Christ (2 Pet. 1:4).
- I have authority as a child of God (Eph. 2:6; Gal. 4:6–7).
- I am a friend of Jesus (John 15:15).
- I have been chosen by Jesus (John 15:16).
- I am loved dearly by God (John 15:13; 16:27; Rom. 5:8; Eph. 3:17–19).
- I am valuable (1 Cor. 6:20).
- I have a mind that is set on God (Col. 3:1–4).
- I have a sound mind (2 Tim. 1:7).

- I am significant (John 15:5).

- I have been chosen by God to bear fruit (John 15:16).

- I have the right to approach God with freedom and confidence (Eph. 3:12).

- I can do all things through Christ who strengthens me (Phil. 4:13).

"If I Help You, How Is That Going to Change Your Life?"

I wouldn't be surprised if by now you're tired of hearing me talk about Dr. Ed Stiles, my manual medicine mentor. But humor me one last time. Let me pass more of his wisdom on to you because it could change your life dramatically for the better.

When Dr. Stiles meets a longtime pain sufferer, he asks, "If I help you, how is that going to change your life?" He gets the patient to think about both positive and negative lifestyle changes that will naturally accompany the healing. And he gets them to think about these things early on in the therapy.

Because of Dr. Stiles's manual treatment paradigm, countless numbers of patients have experienced physical and even emotional healing. Often they get off pain medicine entirely. But on the other hand, that means there is an increase in what others expect of them. The spouse expects more housework and/or sex (if that's a downside to the patient), or friends, family, and coworkers may expect them to meet higher demands.

Or even worse: the patient loses his or her whipping boy. If the patient previously thought, "I'd go back to school and get my degree if it weren't for this back problem," when the back problem resolves, what's stopping him or her from taking that plunge? Now we're down to the real barrier: fear of failure.

Will the patient have to return to work after a long time off? Will he or she lose worker's compensation benefits? Or will he or she lose the excuse to get out of social expectations? There can be very real downsides to "getting well" that offset the benefits in the minds of some people. Believe it or not, it can be scary for patients to face change, even if it's a good change such as reduced pain or increased physical functioning.

That's why Dr. Stiles teaches us to help patients focus on the right things. We tell patients to not necessarily expect to be pain-free but, instead, to look toward increased functioning as they release their physical, emotional, and even spiritual layers of restriction.

Because of the relief we impart to you, can you function better with less pain medicine? Can you tolerate more emotional stress before hurting? Can you sit in the bleachers at your grandson's ball game now when you couldn't previously? Can you now sit in the car for the two-hour trip to visit your sister? These things represent improvement for some patients, even if they don't represent absolute perfection.

Dr. Stiles also helps people focus on their strengths. He routinely says things such as, "Your body has an amazing ability to adapt and change. Your body knows what it needs to do." Or, "Even after all these years, your body can still realize its potential." He's very positive and reminds people of their inborn (and let me add "God-given") ability to heal.

Now let's apply these truths to your life. What will you do with your time when you no longer suffer with irritable bowel syndrome or migraine headaches, or when your addictive, drug-seeking behavior goes away? For that matter, *who will you be* when you're no longer a compulsive shopper, eater, cutter, or workaholic? The capacity is within you to heal from your problem even after all these years, but we need to get your thinking in line with positive, uplifting truth—God's truth.

If on some level you're worried about letting go of the biggest thorn in your side (your pain, addiction, illness, etc.) because of the increased expectations that will be placed on you, stop worrying. You are more than a conqueror through Jesus Christ, and you will be more than strong enough to deal with new pressures that arise.

I hope you see that as encouraging. Neither God nor I promised you'd be perfected at any stage of the game in your physical body. But if you follow the principles in this book, you ought to feel less stress, more peace, and less physical pain along the way as you seek greater and greater levels of Spirit-led healing.

CONCLUSION

A S A CHILD perhaps you believed lies about yourself such as "I'm worthless" or "I'm unlovable" due in part to the lies the accuser told you. And perhaps later in life those beliefs threatened your health, directly or indirectly, by stressing you out and triggering you to reach for false comforters such as food, cigarettes, or drugs and alcohol. Maybe you even experienced pain or illness as a result of those beliefs, as I did.

But now that you've read this book and learned from my patients' real-life experiences, you're different. You understand the importance of shedding the light of God's truth onto those hidden, shameful dark parts of your mind where the lies hide out. Moreover you know how to prayerfully access God's healing truth to replace those lies. You understand the importance of overcoming your barriers to hearing from God and the importance of prayerfully asking the right questions to help you overcome anything that may be blocking you from hearing, feeling, and knowing Him.

You even have new, specific language to use in prayer, as well other tools such as positive language and self-talk exercises, giving God permission to access your imagination, and reciting Scripture and other biblical affirmations out loud. Those tools can come in very handy, especially during times of stress.

Most importantly you have seen what happened to my patients who repented of sin, accepted God's forgiveness, and extended forgiveness to others. Doing these things literally healed my patients' physical problems in certain cases. This result is probably why repenting and extending forgiveness aren't just good ideas from a stress-management point of view. They're also biblical mandates. Without them you cannot achieve the radical well-being God wants you to have in mind, body, and spirit.

As if that wasn't enough practical nuts-and-bolts information to turn your life around, I even told you about two medical diagnoses, myofascial pain syndrome and somatic dysfunction, that could explain a number of your oddball symptoms—the unexplained headaches, spine pain, and even bowel and bladder disturbances. And I told you how to find the best clinicians for treatment of these conditions, right down to website URLs and telling you what to ask the physical therapists' secretaries when you call. Talk about spoon-feeding!

As I close, let me thank you for the time you devoted to reading my book. And let me pray that God blesses you with divine understanding of what parts of this book relate to you and what parts you can ignore (at least for now). In addition I pray God gives you the grace and mercy to eat the fish I provided despite any bones I inadvertently left behind.

Keep in mind that these "healer" and "author" roles are evolving journeys for me too! I honestly don't believe I have all the answers you need. God Himself is the ultimate authority regarding what ails you in your emotions and your spirit. So prayerfully run everything I said past Him if you have questions. And don't forget to check with your personal physician regarding the medical information I presented. Only he or she (inspired by God, I hope) can know what part of this information, if any, applies in your situation.

Your journey to wholeness and healing is a lifelong process, not an instantaneous fix. Hold firm to your Christian belief system, and God will bless you abundantly, not only in terms of your physical health but also with overall peace and joy that surpasses all understanding.

Appendix A

PRAYING FOR EMOTIONAL HEALING

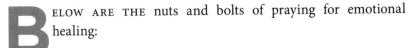ELOW ARE THE nuts and bolts of praying for emotional healing:

- Pray daily. It's your source of motivation and strength. I'm reminded of a quote attributed to author Zig Ziglar, "People often say that motivation doesn't last. Well, neither does bathing—that's why we recommend it daily."[1]

- Pray about whether you may need formal Christian counseling or formal medical supervision. If you decide to actually implement my ideas, err on the side of being cautious and seek counseling from a licensed Christian therapist, physician, or secular counselor (and then pray for your counselor to help you)!

- You may decide to model some of your prayers after the Lord's Prayer. Notice that it offers praise to God, submission to Him, request for provision, a request for and an offering of forgiveness, a request for strength to withstand temptation, and deliverance from evil.

- Pray for God to help you recognize, capture, and name your difficult emotions in case you have trouble identifying them.

- Pray for God to help you realize which emotions trigger you to reach for false comforters. Are you triggered to eat by fear (which is often disguised as worry, anxiety, anger, perfectionism, workaholism, or being overcontrolling of yourself or others)? Or are you triggered by depression and dissatisfaction with yourself and others?

- Ask God to help you isolate the specific past emotional injuries that underlie your emotional triggers.

- Ask God to bring you these memories, either through images in your mind's eye or maybe through physical sensations or mere thoughts that pop into your head.

- Ask God for mercy as He reveals these past memories to you, so you can take it slowly and not be overwhelmed. Even if you don't ask, He gives you only what you can handle.

Specific Prayers

Prayer for emotional healing for weight loss

Dear Lord, cut the strings that connect my emotions with the way I eat. Free me from the triggers that manipulate me. Restore me to health in all dimensions—in mind, body, and spirit. Amen.

Prayer for receiving forgiveness

Dear Lord, forgive my sins, past, present, and future, those that I'm aware of and those that I'm unaware of, including the sins of my entire bloodline, which have led to my disordered eating and other health problems. Help me to feel Your forgiveness in the depths of my being. Amen.

Prayer for extending forgiveness

Lord, I fully and completely release [fill in the person's name] to you and I forgive [him or her] for what [he or she] did to me. I expect no apology or explanation from this person. I cancel [his or her] debt entirely, with nothing expected in return. Thank You for freeing me from the burden of unforgiveness. Amen.

Prayer for surrender

Dear Lord, I surrender my whole mind, body, and soul to You. Please transform me the way You promised in Romans 12:1–2, so I can feel the fruit of Your Spirit—peace, wholeness, and joy. Amen.

Prayer for connection of feeling and right thinking

Lord, I believe You when You say I am the apple of Your eye. I believe You when You say I'm washed clean by the blood of Jesus. I believe You when You say I can do great things in Your name. Now, help me to feel this truth as deeply as I know it. Amen.

Prayer for healing of emotions

Lord, show me Your healing truth in my innermost places so I can feel peace, joy, and gladness. Let the light of Your truth bring wholeness and balance to my being. Amen.

Prayer for inner peace

Lord, search me and help me identify the thoughts and emotions that rob me of peace. Help me to reject those thoughts and refocus on what is right and good, according to Your Word. Amen.

Prayer for right thinking

Lord, examine my thinking at all levels, from the conscious to the subconscious, and purge me of the darkness, lies, and wrong thinking that corrupt my emotions. Amen.

Prayer of authority over false emotions

By the shed blood of Jesus I command all forms of darkness, negativity, lies, disorder, and disease to leave my emotional and physical being and go straight to the foot of Jesus. Amen.

Prayer for release from generational oppression

Lord, release me from the consequences of the sins of my bloodline. Wash me clean of any and all oppressive forces that are in my family lineage, past, present, or future. Amen.

Appendix B

SCRIPTURE FOR SELF-TALK AND MEDITATION

Instead of the lies that leave you feeling	Believe the truth
Fearful	Fear is not from God (2 Tim. 1:7).
Worried	God gives peace (1 Pet. 5:7; Phil. 4:6–7).
Lost	God directs my steps (Prov. 3:5–6).
Stupid	God gives me wisdom (1 Cor. 1:30).
Unattractive	God makes me attractive (Ezek. 16:14).
Worthless	I was bought at a high price (1 Cor. 6:20).
Unwanted	God chose me on purpose (Eph. 1:4).
Weighed down with burdens	God takes my burdens (Ps. 55:22).
Out of control	The Spirit rules over the flesh (Rom. 8:9).
Abandoned	God is always with me (Heb. 13:5).
Confused	God gives me a sound mind (2 Tim. 1:7).
Unlovable	God loves me (John 3:16; Rom. 8:39).
Shameful	God doesn't condemn me (Rom. 8:1).
Bad	Only God is good (Luke 18:19).
Guilty	I am blameless (Col. 1:22).
Like it's all your fault	God freed me from blame (Eph. 1:4).

Invisible, unimportant	God sees me (1 Cor. 8:3).
Like you don't have what you need	God supplies my needs (Phil. 4:19).
Inept	God makes me able (2 Cor. 3:5).
Unforgivable	God forgives all (Ps. 103:8–10).
Weak	Christ strengthens me (Phil. 4:13).
Dirty	Jesus's blood cleanses (Heb. 9:14).
Like you don't have enough faith	God gave everyone faith (Rom. 12:3).
Like it's impossible	I can do all things (Luke 18:27).
Lacking the energy to do it	God gives me rest (Matt. 11:28–30).
Like you can't do it	I *can* (Phil. 4:13, 2 Cor. 9:8; Rom. 8:37).
Like it's not worth it	It is worth it (Rom. 8:28).
Like you can't be forgiven	I am forgiven (1 John 1:9, Rom. 8:1).
Wanting to be perfect	I don't have to be perfect (2 Cor. 12:9–10).

Other faulty thoughts and emotions	**The truth that refutes the lie**
_____	_____
_____	_____
_____	_____
_____	_____
_____	_____
_____	_____
_____	_____
_____	_____
_____	_____
_____	_____
_____	_____

Scriptures for Emotional Healing

You intended to harm me, but God intended it for good to accomplish what is now being done, the saving of many lives.

—GENESIS 50:20

I sought the LORD, and he answered me; he delivered me from all my fears.

—PSALM 34:4

The LORD is close to the brokenhearted and saves those who are crushed in spirit. The righteous may have many troubles, but the LORD delivers them from them all.

—PSALM 34:18–19

Surely you desire truth in the inner parts; you teach me wisdom in the inmost place.

—PSALM 51:6

"Because he loves me," says the LORD, "I will rescue him; I will protect him, for he acknowledges my name."

—PSALM 91:14

Search me, O God, and know my heart; test me and know my anxious thoughts. See if there is any offensive way in me, and lead me in the way everlasting.

—PSALM 139:23–24

Surely he took up our infirmities and carried our sorrows, yet we considered him stricken by God, smitten by him, and afflicted. But he was pierced for our transgressions, he was crushed for our iniquities; the punishment that brought us peace was on him, and by his wounds we are healed.

—ISAIAH 53:4–5

If my people, who are called by my name, will humble themselves and pray and seek my face and turn from their wicked ways, then will I hear from heaven and will forgive their sin and will heal their land.

—2 Chronicles 7:14

Heal me, Lord, and I will be healed; save me and I will be saved, for you are the one I praise.

—Jeremiah 17:14

"But I will restore you to health and heal your wounds," declares the Lord, "because you are called an outcast, Zion for whom no one cares."

—Jeremiah 30:17

Jesus went throughout Galilee, teaching in their synagogues, proclaiming the good news of the kingdom, and healing every disease and sickness among the people.

—Matthew 4:23

When evening came, many who were demon-possessed were brought to him, and he drove out the spirits with a word and healed all the sick. This was to fulfill what was spoken through the prophet Isaiah: "He took up our infirmities and bore our diseases."

—Matthew 8:16–17

Heal the sick, raise the dead, cleanse those who have leprosy, drive out demons. Freely you have received, freely give.

—Matthew 10:8

I tell you the truth, whatever you bind on earth will be bound in heaven, and whatever you loose on earth will be loosed in heaven. Again, I tell you that if two of you on earth agree about anything you ask for, it will be done for you by my Father in heaven.

—Matthew 18:18–19

Jesus replied, "I tell you the truth, if you have faith and do not doubt, not only can you do what was done to the fig tree, but also you can say to this mountain, 'Go, throw yourself into the sea,' and it will be done. If you believe, you will receive whatever you ask for in prayer."

—MATTHEW 21:21–22

I tell you the truth, if anyone says to this mountain, "Go, throw yourself into the sea," and does not doubt in his heart but believes that what he says will happen, it will be done for him. Therefore I tell you, whatever you ask for in prayer, believe that you have received it, and it will be yours.

—MARK 11:23–24

The Spirit of the Lord is on me, because he has anointed me to preach good news to the poor. He has sent me to proclaim freedom for the prisoners and recovery of sight for the blind, to release the oppressed.

—LUKE 4:18

Peace I leave with you; my peace I give you. I do not give to you as the world gives. Do not let your hearts be troubled and do not be afraid.

—JOHN 14:27

For this people's heart has become calloused; they hardly hear with their ears, and they have closed their eyes. Otherwise they might see with their eyes, hear with their ears, understand with their hearts and turn, and I would heal them.

—ACTS 28:27

Therefore, there is now no condemnation for those who are in Christ Jesus.

—ROMANS 8:1

For you did not receive a spirit that makes you a slave again to fear, but you received the Spirit of sonship. And by him we cry, "Abba, Father." The Spirit himself testifies with our spirit that we are God's children.

—ROMANS 8:15–16

And we know that in all things God works for the good of those who love him, who have been called according to his purpose.

—ROMANS 8:28

The weapons we fight with are not the weapons of the world. On the contrary, they have divine power to demolish strongholds. We demolish arguments and every pretension that sets itself up against the knowledge of God, and we take captive every thought to make it obedient to Christ.

—2 CORINTHIANS 10:4–5

But he said to me, "My grace is sufficient for you, for my power is made perfect in weakness." Therefore I will boast all the more gladly about my weaknesses, so that Christ's power may rest on me.

—2 CORINTHIANS 12:9

Do not be anxious about anything, but in everything, by prayer and petition, with thanksgiving, present your requests to God. And the peace of God, which transcends all understanding, will guard your hearts and your minds in Christ Jesus.

—PHILIPPIANS 4:6–7

And my God will meet all your needs according to his glorious riches in Christ Jesus.

—PHILIPPIANS 4:19

Therefore confess your sins to each other and pray for each other so that you may be healed. The prayer of a righteous person is powerful and effective.

—JAMES 5:16

He himself bore our sins in his body on the tree, so that we might die to sins and live for righteousness; by his wounds you have been healed.

—1 PETER 2:24

And the God of all grace, who called you to his eternal glory in Christ, after you have suffered a little while, will himself restore you and make you strong, firm and steadfast.

—1 PETER 5:10

They overcame him by the blood of the Lamb and by the word of their testimony; they did not love their lives so much as to shrink from death.

—REVELATION 12:11

NOTES

Chapter 2
Trace Your Triggers

1. Quinn Schipper, *Trading Faces* (Stillwater, OK: New Forums Press, 2005).

Chapter 3
Stress Less, Betty

1. Bruce McEwen, "Allostasis and Allostatic Load: Implications for Neuropsychopharmacology," *Neuropsychopharmacology* 22, no. 2 (February 2000), 108–124.

2. J. Schofferman, D. Anderson, R. Hines, G. Smith, and A. White, "Childhood Psychological Trauma Correlates With Unsuccessful Lumbar Spine Surgery," *Spine* 17, suppl 6 (June 1992): S138–S144.

Chapter 5
New Hope for Pain Sufferers

1. "MET For The Upper Half," Mercy Hospital Spine Center, Oklahoma City, December 4, 2010.

2. Ibid.

3. In conversation with Dr. Ed Stiles, September 2012, Mercy Hospital, Oklahoma City, OK. The course was called "Functional Indirect Techniques."

Chapter 6
Sometimes Your Senses Lie

1. Candace Pert, *Molecules of Emotion* (New York: Scribner, 1997).

Chapter 7
The Accuser

1. *Avatar*, directed by James Cameron (Los Angeles, CA: Twentieth Century Fox Home Entertainment, 2010), DVD.

2. *Family Matters* (Burbank, CA: Warner Bros. Television Distribution, 1989–1998).

Chapter 8
You Are Delightful

1. Patrick Morley, *The Man in the Mirror* (Grand Rapids, MI: Zondervan, 2011), 105–106. Viewed at Google Books.

2. *Enjoying Everyday Life*, July 7, 2010, parts 1-3, http://www.youtube
.com/watch?v=Syxc4o4O47Q (accessed September 18, 2012).

3. Oswald Chambers, *My Utmost for His Highest*, "June 13," (Uhrichs-
ville, OH: Barbour Books, 2000).

Chapter 10
Taking Control

1. Podcast-Directory-Co-Uk, "Dr. Mike Murdock Wisdom Teachings,"
http://www.podcast-directory.co.uk/episodes/wisdom-key-10-your-focus
-decides-your-feelings-14739732.html (accessed September 18, 2012).

2. Henriët van Middendorp, Mark A. Lumley, Johannes W. G. Jacobs,
Johannes W. J. Bijlsma, and Rinie Geenen, "The Effects of Anger and Sadness on Clinical Pain Reports and Experimentally-Induced Pain Thresholds
in Women With and Without Fibromyalgia," *Arthritis Care and Research*
62, no. 10 (October 2010): http://onlinelibrary.wiley.com/doi/10.1002/
acr.20230/full (accessed September 18, 2012).

3. Michael L. Slepian, E. J. Masicampo, Negin R. Toosi, and Nalini
Ambady, "The Physical Burdens of Secrecy," *Journal of Experimental Psychology* (March 5, 2012), http://ambadylab.stanford.edu/pubs/Slepian
-Masicampo-Toosi-Ambady_Physical-Burdens-of-Secrecy_in-press_JEPG
.pdf (accessed September 18, 2012).

4. Ibid.

5. Alison L. Hill, David G. Rand, Martin A. Nowak, and Nicholas A.
Christakis, "Emotions as Infectious Diseases in a Large Social Network:
The SISa Model," *Proceedings for the Royal Society* B (July 7, 2010): http://
rspb.royalsocietypublishing.org/content/early/2010/07/03/rspb.2010.1217
(accessed September 18, 2012).

Chapter 12
Have No Fear!

1. *Star Wars: Episode I—The Phantom Menace*, directed by George
Lucas (Los Angeles, CA: Twentieth Century Fox Home Entertainment,
1999), DVD.

2. National Institute on Drug Abuse, "Research Reports: Prescription Drugs: Abuse and Addiction," http://tinyurl.com/9qqjhkg (accessed
October 3, 2012).

Chapter 13
Power Plays

1. C. S. Lewis, *Mere Christianity* (New York: HarperOne, 2001), 122.
Viewed at Google Books.

Chapter 14
Reject Perfectionism

1. As quoted in Stan Guthrie, *All That Jesus Asks* (Grand Rapids, MI: Baker Books, 2010), 113. Viewed at Google Books.

Chapter 16
Filtering Out Lies in Advertising

1. Mike Bernie, "Arnold Launches 'Hershey's Pure' Campaign," http://www.adweek.com/news/advertising-branding/arnold-launches-hersheys-pure-campaign-96533 (accessed September 19, 2012).

2. Esther K. Papies, Wolfgang Stroebe, and Henk Aarts, "Who Likes It More? Restrained Eaters' Implicit Attitudes Towards Food," *Appetite* 53, no. 1 (August 2009): 279–287; http://tinyurl.com/8p7mnnp (accessed September 19, 2012).

3. Steve Helling, "Nia Vardalos Explains How She Lost 40 Lbs.," *People*, http://www.people.com/people/article/0,,20276444,00.html (accessed September 19, 2012).

4. American Dairy Association, http://ilovecheese.com/ (accessed September 19, 2012).

5. LiveDash.com, *Piers Morgan Tonight*, Monday, February 21, 2011, CNN transcript, http://www.livedash.com/transcript/piers_morgan_tonight/49/CNN/Monday_February_21_2011/563295/ (accessed September 19, 2012).

6. Golden Corral, "About Us," http://www.goldencorral.com/about/ (accessed September 19, 2012).

7. Jeff Bailey, "Reinventing Applebee's," *Forbes*, http://www.forbes.com/2009/12/02/restaurant-business-applebees-ihop-julia-stewart.html (accessed September 19, 2012).

8. Burger King, "Our History," http://www.bk.com/en/us/company-info/about-bk.html (accessed September 19, 2012).

9. I personally saw this billboard.

10. iVillage.com, "McDonald's: Make Up Your Own Mind," http://www.ivillage.co.uk/mcdonalds-make-your-own-mind/78767 (accessed September 19, 2012).

11. YouTube.com, "Dunkin' Donuts | 'Tractor Beam'" http://www.youtube.com/watch?v=QOydrJgmO_k (accessed September 19, 2012).

12. YouTube.com, "McDonald's You Deserve a Break Today," http://www.youtube.com/watch?v=BqRH8wEsaVQ (accessed September 19, 2012).

13. Hersheys.com, "KitKat," http://www.hersheys.com/kitkat.aspx (accessed September 19, 2012).

14. Olive Garden, "When You're Here, You're Family," http://www .olivegarden.com/ (accessed September 19, 2012).

15. Wikipedia.com, "Pringles," http://en.wikipedia.org/wiki/Pringles (accessed September 19, 2012).

16. YouTube.com, "Kellogg's Special K: Chocolatey Delight," http://www .youtube.com/watch?v=IJTV65pSweo (accessed September 19, 2012).

Chapter 19
Introduction to Inner Healing

1. Theophostic Prayer Ministry, "Theophostic Prayer Ministry Session Guidelines," http://theophostic.com/guidelines.aspx (accessed October 3, 2012).

Chapter 23
Your True Identity

1. Popular quotation attributed to Blaise Pascal. "Inspirational Quotes," Beliefnet.com, http://www.beliefnet.com/Quotes/Evangelical/B/Blaise -Pascal/Not-Only-Do-We-Not-Know-God-Except-Through-Jesus-C.aspx (accessed September 21, 2012).

2. *Star Trek: The Original Series*, "The Doomsday Machine" directed by Marc Daniels, original air date October 20, 1967, CBS (Culver City, CA: Desilu Studios, 1967).

3. Craig Groeschel, *Chazown* (Colorado Springs, CO: Multnomah Books, 2010).

Appendix A

1. ThinkExist.com, "Zig Ziglar quotes," http://thinkexist.com/quotation/ people_often_say_that_motivation_doesn-t_last/145449.html (accessed September 24, 2012).

ABOUT THE AUTHOR

I INVITE YOU TO connect with me and learn about my new books on Facebook under Doctor Rita's Author Page, on Twitter under @RitaHancockMD, and via my websites www.RadicalWell-Being .com, www.TheEdenDiet.com, and www.RitaHancock.com.

INDEX

A

abandon (-ed, -ment) 3–4, 12–13, 16, 24, 40, 62, 77, 85, 120, 124, 127, 133–134, 143, 145, 153–155, 199, 202, 248

abuse (-ed, -s) 6, 9, 16–17, 37, 65, 77, 85, 99, 124, 128, 155–156, 171, 178–179, 186, 197, 199, 202

   physical, -ly 24, 61, 66

   sexual, -ly 12

   verbal, -ly 80

abuser 210, 227

accuser 19, 27, 73–76, 79, 81, 83, 86, 88, 92, 95–96, 100–101, 121, 152, 155, 208–209, 218, 227, 231, 242

addiction(s) 5, 48, 77, 87, 112, 127, 146, 155, 171, 178, 228, 240

addictive behaviors 240

affirmation(s) 138, 225, 227, 229–231, 242

alcoholic(s) 40, 99, 147

Alcoholics Anonymous 146

allostasis 23–24

allostatic load 24

alprazolam 22

American Academy of Osteopathy 55

American Academy of Physical Medicine and Rehabilitation 51

American Association of Christian Counselors 213

amitriptyline 22

anger 8, 33, 65, 74, 97, 106, 115–116, 126, 137, 149, 156, 171, 182, 184–185, 193, 203, 207, 224, 228, 244

anorexia 143

anterior cingulate gyrus 44

antidepressant 22

anxiety 4–5, 11, 20–23, 48, 76–77, 98, 101, 123–128, 130, 133, 136–137, 147, 149, 153–154, 183, 191–193, 203, 207, 224, 228, 244

arrhythmias 36

arthritis 21, 53, 125, 140

Arthritis Care and Research 106

autoimmune disease 173

B

barrier(s) 9, 18, 28, 42, 55, 69, 82, 92–93, 102, 139, 167, 177, 184, 187, 201, 205, 218, 228, 239, 242

binge(s) 31, 40, 43, 79, 136

bipolar disorder 178, 181

bitterness 18, 33, 74, 154, 171, 179, 185, 220

brain fog 52

bursitis 136

C

caffeine 34–35

cancer 11, 31, 34, 173

carpal tunnel syndrome 121

cerebral area 44

cerebral cortex 44

Chambers, Oswald 89

chiropractic medicine 57–58

Christian counselor 5, 109, 130, 192–193, 198, 200, 212–213

Christian Counselors Directory 213

chronic dieting, dieters   99, 159–160

chronic pain   99

compulsive eater   98, 159, 240

compulsive eating disorder   86,

condemnation   90–91, 95, 173, 176,
   230, 238, 252

conversion disorder(s)   38, 48

counseling   4, 8, 67, 97–98, 193, 197,
   200, 205–206, 212–213, 234, 244

   Christian   97, 134, 192–193, 244

   emotional   39, 192

   psychological   45, 174

counter-stimulation   225–226

craniosacral OMM   56–57

cutting   8, 40

D

deliverance   198, 210–212, 234, 244

depression   5, 15, 20–22, 43, 48, 65,
   101, 115, 130, 175, 178, 184, 193, 203,
   224, 228, 232, 245

DeSilva, Dawna   201

diabetes   136

dissociative identity disorder   203

divorce(d)   4, 6, 16, 43, 46, 153–154,
   178, 208

doctors of osteopathy (DO)   46, 54,
   56, 63, 234

dysfunctional   125, 150, 155, 164, 181–
   182, 196, 221

E

eating disorder(s)   1–2, 8, 48, 86, 88,
   120, 161

Eden Diet, The   1, 115, 159

egocentric   77

Eldredge, John and Stasi   87

electrical nerve test(s), -ing   121, 204

electrical stimulation treament   61

electrodiagnostic studies
   (EMGs)   50

embryo(s)   89–96, 101, 209

EMDR   212

emotional

   eating   4, 21–22, 99, 120, 135, 224

   healing   12, 18–19, 87, 150, 216,
      233, 236, 239, 244–245, 250

   tension   33, 60, 63, 141, 215

Enjoying Everyday Life   87

F

facial tics   41

false

   belief(s)   5, 7, 13, 16, 19, 157, 193

   comforter(s)   5, 8–9, 12, 16, 27,
      64–66, 68, 76–78, 95, 106, 114,
      116, 119–121, 124, 127, 129–130,
      133, 137–139, 146–147, 149, 152,
      157, 159, 193, 224, 228, 230, 242,
      244

   emotion(s)   229–231, 234, 246

   memories   197

fear(s)   4, 8, 11–12, 16–18, 24, 27,
      35–36, 64–66, 74, 76, 79, 116, 123–
      131, 137, 139, 141, 143, 145, 156, 177,
      191–192, 207, 219, 228, 244, 248,
      250, 252

   of abandonment   13, 24–25, 120,
      145, 154–155

   of death   156

   of discomfort   18

   of failure   239

of feeling   129

of pain   130

of Y2K   25

react to   123

fetus(es)   92–96, 101, 209, 217, 236

fibromyalgia   11, 20–21, 26, 34, 44, 47, 53–54, 106, 137

fight-or-flight   25

forgive(-n, -ness)   7, 9–10, 18–19, 25, 60, 69, 78, 97, 102, 117, 122, 139, 148, 154, 157, 162, 172, 176–179, 181–187, 193, 201, 207, 209–210, 219–220, 228, 230, 233, 238, 242, 244–245, 249, 251

frontal lobe   44

Furtick, Steven   110

G

GABA (gamma-aminobutyric acid)   45

generational

bondage   228

curse(s)   169, 171, 203

guilt(y)   4, 15–16, 25, 27, 74–75, 78, 80, 84, 119, 124, 139, 156, 163, 168, 171, 175, 180, 183–185, 187, 230, 248

H

heart

attack(s)   41, 52, 171

failure   36

herniated disk   31

high velocity low amplitude (HVLA) techniques   55–56

hippocampus   45

hoarding   40

hurt inner child   97

hydrocodone   33

hypochondriasis   48

I

inadequate   4, 7–8, 99, 142, 237

injections   20, 23, 26, 32, 78, 109, 179, 204, 232

trigger point injections   20, 50–51, 155, 215

inner

child   12, 19, 97, 207–210, 215–217, 220, 227

healing   9, 153, 191–199, 201–207, 210–212, 218–219

insomnia   20, 33–34, 40, 48

insular cortex   44

International Society of Deliverance Ministers (ISDM)   197, 212

interstitial cystitis   47

in vivo exposure   130

irritable bowel syndrome (IBS)   20, 26, 47, 137, 153, 224, 240

L

Language of Forgiveness, The   219

lap-band procedure   136

latissimus dorsi   53

Lewis, C. S.   137

limbic

forebrain   44

system   44, 63–65

lupus   21, 49, 53

M

Man in the Mirror, The   83

manual

   medicine   9, 21, 24, 26, 54, 56, 58, 201, 204, 206, 239. *See also* osteopathic manual medicine (OMM)

   PT   56–57

McAfee, Robert   22

McEwen, Bruce   24

medulla   44

memory (-ies)   12, 17, 19, 24, 26, 45, 61–62, 64–66, 85–86, 88, 91, 97, 132, 153, 156, 192, 194, 198–200, 202, 205, 208, 225, 227, 245

meningitis   38

mental illness   76, 155, 172, 178, 181–182, 198

Meyer, Joyce   87

migraine(s)   20–21, 26, 41, 137, 240

Molecules of Emotion   64

multiple sclerosis (MS)   78

Murdock, Mike   105

muscle

   disorders   121

   spasms   11, 36, 141

myofascial pain syndrome (MPS)   48–51, 53–54, 58–59, 243

N

National Christian Counselors Association   213

negative emotion(s)   12, 33, 67–68, 79, 130, 156–157, 171, 193, 222, 225, 228–229

neglect (-ed)   17, 85, 142, 199

nerve(s)   5, 38, 44–45, 47, 49, 121, 127, 157, 170, 185, 204, 225, 234

neuroplasticity   45

neurosis   48

nonnarcotic numbing medicine   20, 50

North American Academy of Manual Medicine (NAAMM)   50

O

occupational therapy   39

opiate   64

osteopath   234

osteopathic manual medicine (OMM)   20–21, 26, 32–33, 46, 50–59, 61, 67, 107, 140, 153, 155, 174, 179, 196, 201, 204–206, 215–216, 234. *See also* manual medicine

P

pain management   1, 38, 48–49, 51, 63–64, 125, 127–128, 130, 149, 196, 201, 204–205, 222, 225

pain medicine   33, 127, 129, 239–240

panic

   attack(s)   43, 66, 136

   disorders   48

paralysis   40, 175

paralyzed   38–39

perfection (-ism, -ist)   2, 99, 140–148, 228, 240, 244

periaqueductal gray matter (PAG)   44

personality disorder(s)   48, 124

Pert, Candace   64

physiatrist(s)   49–51

physical

    therapist(s)   24, 26, 56–57, 234, 243

    therapy   9, 31–32, 38–40, 50, 56–57, 61

physical medicine and rehabilitation (PM&R)   49

Pope, Ross   59

prenatal

    communication   92

    regressions   97

pride   74, 77, 80–81, 101, 127, 137

protective postures   37, 46

pseudo-addiction   129–130

psychology   4, 9, 114–115, 197, 201

psychosis   48

Q

quadratus lumborum   53

R

receptor(s)   64

referred pain   49

reframing   97, 193

rejection   120, 151, 154

repressed   17, 20–21, 27, 64

resentment   18, 182, 184–185

restless leg syndrome   35, 41, 48

restrained eaters   159–160, 162

restriction(s)   18, 31, 52, 56–58, 240

rheumatoid arthritis   21, 53

rheumatologic disorders   21, 53

right thinking   111, 246

rostral ventral nucleus (RVM)   44

rotator cuff   215

S

sacral bone   53

sacroiliac joints (SI joints)   51

Sale, Micha   26

Schipper, Quinn   17, 202–203, 207–208, 219

seizure(s)   41, 132

self-

    centered (-ness)   77, 112, 126

    condemnation   14, 79, 175

    discipline   107, 111

    esteem   2–4, 8, 67–68, 77, 80, 88, 90, 99, 101, 119, 126, 141, 144, 151, 207

    judgment   14, 80

    talk   224, 226–228, 242, 248

sequencing   50–51, 56–57

Serenity Prayer   146

serotonin   34

sexual abuse   16, 85, 155, 202

sexually abused   6, 37, 77

shame   3, 25, 74, 76, 85, 93, 96–97, 116, 119, 156, 175, 224, 230

shingles   41, 47, 137

SI joint pain   51

sleepwalking   41, 48

Smith, Ed M.   199

soft tissue injections   20

soft tissue "trigger point" injections   20

somatic dysfunction (SD)   48–49, 51–54, 56, 58–59, 243

somatization disorder   48

somato emotional releases   62

somatoform disorders   48

somatovisceral reflexes   52

soul ties   177, 203

Sozo   197, 201–202, 205

SOZO Ministry   201–202

speech disorder   39–40

spinal cortisone shots   31

spinal injections   78, 179

spiritual gifts   235–237

steroid(s)   32, 136, 206

Stiles, Ed   21–25, 45–46, 50–51, 56, 58, 63, 239–240

stress   2, 4–5, 16, 20–28, 31–33, 36, 38–44, 46–48, 62, 95, 99–100, 105, 113, 127, 140–141, 151–152, 154–155, 168–170, 172, 175, 179, 185, 187, 215, 219, 222, 225, 227, 229, 233, 234, 240–242

stress eat (-ing)   26, 62, 65, 75, 187

stress-induced illnesses   11, 20–22, 27, 32, 36, 41, 47–48, 62, 100, 109, 137

stress urticaria   20

strife   2, 149, 151–152, 171, 221–222

subconscious (-ly)   3, 5, 26, 36–37, 40, 43, 46, 48, 77, 79, 85, 90, 100, 115, 119, 123, 132–133, 138, 145, 159, 246

subconscious memories   62

T

Takotsubo cardiomyopathy   36, 109

TENS unit   225

Theophostic   197, 199–200, 202, 205

Theophostic Prayer Ministry (TPM)   199–200

tissue tension   23, 33, 52, 206

Trading Faces   17, 202–203, 208, 219

transcutaneous electricl nerve stimulation (TENS)   225

Travell, Janet   50–51

trichotillomania   40

U

ulcer(s)   20, 26, 40, 47, 113

unforgiveness   28, 60, 102, 167, 170–171, 177, 179, 184–185, 187, 210, 220, 222, 245

V

vertebra prominens   43

viscerosomatic reflexes   52

W

Wallnau, Lance   115

Williams, Marleen   120, 161

workaholic, workaholism   2, 143, 240, 244

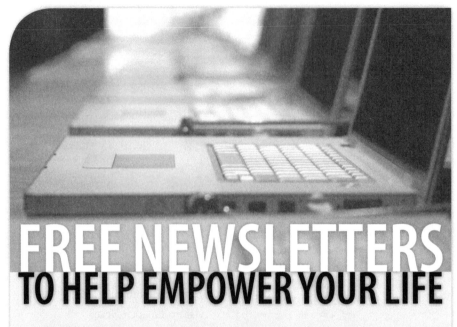

FREE NEWSLETTERS
TO HELP EMPOWER YOUR LIFE

Why subscribe today?

- ❏ **DELIVERED DIRECTLY TO YOU.** All you have to do is open your inbox and read.

- ❏ **EXCLUSIVE CONTENT.** We cover the news overlooked by the mainstream press.

- ❏ **STAY CURRENT.** Find the latest court rulings, revivals, and cultural trends.

- ❏ **UPDATE OTHERS.** Easy to forward to friends and family with the click of your mouse.

CHOOSE THE E-NEWSLETTER THAT INTERESTS YOU MOST:

- Christian news
- Daily devotionals
- Spiritual empowerment
- And much, much more

SIGN UP AT: **http://freenewsletters.charismamag.com**

8178